Refined to Real Food

Moving Your Family Toward
Healthier, Wholesome Eating

D0962716

Refined to Real Food

Moving Your Family Toward Healthier, Wholesome Eating

Allison Anneser
with Sara Thyr, ND

J. N. Townsend Publishing
Exeter, New Hampshire
2005

Second Printing, 2006.

Cover design by Joyce Weston.

Published by

PublishingWorks, Inc.

J. N. Townsend Publishing

60 Winter Street

Exeter, NH 03833

800/333-9883

www.publishingworks.com

Ordering information from:

Revolution Booksellers, LLC

1-800-REV-6603

www.revolutionbooksellers.com

Library of Congress Cataloging-in-Publication Data

Anneser, Allison.

Refined to real food: moving your family towards healthier, wholesome eating / by Allison Anneser, with Sara Thyr.

p. cm.

Includes bibliographical references and index.

ISBN 1-880158-48-5

1. Nutrition. 2. Food habits. 3. Family—Nutrition. 4. Natural foods. 5. Cookery (Natural foods) I. Thry, Sara. II. Title

3657   4845   10/07

RA784.A538 2004

613.2—dc22   2004063657

ISBN: 1-880158-48-5

$15.95

Acknowledgements

I would like to thank Sara Thyr, ND for serving as nutritional consultant for this book. Her endless expertise, encouragement, and faith in this project made it enjoyable as well as valuable. I would also like to thank other professionals for their feedback and nutritional guidance: Stacey Gillespie, Cynthia Gossler, LJSCW, Tanya Renner, Jeffrey Scott Sullender, Ph.D., CCN, and Gail Vanark, ARNP.

The following people provided helpful advice and honest opinions: Camille Campbell, Michelle Castell, Karen Cerato, Jennifer Costas, Kathy Drury, Lisa Eastland, Kathleen Farwell, Pixie Frank, Anne Gould, Victoria Groves, Sarah May, Kathleen Mello, Jennifer Metcalf, Erin Moskun, Leona Palmer, Joanne Pomeranz, and Chandra Simonds. A special thanks to Virginia B. Martin and Chef Eric Sanford for reviewing recipes and to Jeremy Townsend and Linda Chestney for guiding this project to completion.

And last, but not least, I would like to thank my wonderful family: my parents, Judy and Rod Reck, my patient children, Grace and Scott, and, especially, my supportive husband, Doug. You're the best!

Table of Contents

Table of Tables

Foreword

Sara Thyr

When Allison approached me about her idea for this book I was thrilled. So many patients come into my practice with health problems as a result of poor nutrition. They experience infertility, diabetes, high blood pressure and many other issues. They want to make changes in their diet knowing that it will benefit their health, but don't know how to start. Finally, a resource has been created that people can utilize to improve their own health and the health of their family. This book is not about radical change or doing it all at once. It is about taking small steps; adding more healthful foods at your own pace, whether it is once a week or once a month, but making permanent changes that will last a lifetime.

As a health professional, I often add nutritional supplements or herbs to assist in restoring a client's health, but nearly everyone will see improved health by eating a whole foods diet. In fact, the people in my practice who have experienced the most dramatic changes are those who made a commitment to eat more healthfully. They became empowered by their success and the ability to improve their health with such a simple concept.

While eating whole foods may sound easy, putting this concept into practice may be challenging, especially if you are just starting out. This is where *Refined to Real Food* can help you make the transition. Every meal, every snack, every sip of a beverage is a fresh opportunity to change your body's biochemistry and bring back your vitality and health.

It is important to note that you don't have to do everything at once. Make the changes that are manageable and realistic for you now. Add new foods gradually and enjoy the delicious qualities of each one. Be constant but flexible…keep trying even after giving in to fast food or a more refined meal. Soon you will discover that you feel healthier and experience less illness and disease. These changes will permeate the core of how your family views food. *Believe* that you can make changes and you *will*.

This book is a book for every day. It is a book for life. It is so helpful and inspiring you will want to leave it out on your kitchen table. Healthier eating is a journey and a process. Most likely, it is the most important one you will ever take. As you make healthful changes, you will inspire others to do the same.

Bon appétit! And bon voyage!

Preface

I was trying to eat healthily. I ate baby carrots with my lunch and had an occasional salad-in-the-bag with dinner. I bought low-fat products, although they were high in sugar. I bought sugar-free products, but they were high in fat. I tried counting calories and cutting carbohydrates, but neither lasted.

I was feeling fine. I had a few colds and illnesses, but who hasn't? I was tired, but who wasn't? I could afford to lose a few pounds, but who couldn't? Then I had problems becoming pregnant. After initial infertility treatments proved unsuccessful, a friend suggested I see a certified clinical nutritionist (CCN).

"I believe in the intelligence of the body," the nutritionist said at my first visit. "If you're not getting pregnant, what do you think your body is trying to tell you?" I didn't know what to say. I had never thought this way before, so he said it for me.

"Maybe your body isn't a healthy place to support new life." It was hard to hear, but true. A few tests confirmed that I was low on almost every essential nutrient my body needed (and totally devoid of some) and high on a few toxin scales. I decided to take a hard look at my eating habits, educate myself, and make changes.

I read, researched, returned to the nutritionist, and began learning to cook. I had little faith that changing my diet would have any impact, but made the commitment to eating more healthful foods. After a few days, I had more energy. After a few weeks, I lost weight and managed to avoid a cold going around. After a few months, I was pregnant. Like many health problems, my infertility was nutritionally based. We are what we eat. To be healthy, experience less illness and disease, and live longer and happier lives, we need to eat real foods. *Refined to Real Food* is the book I wish I had had when I finally decided to become serious about eating right. Anyone can eat healthier foods for a few months, but I wanted to eat this way for the rest of my life. Not only was I searching for information about the most nutritious foods, I wanted to know how to incorporate these foods into my diet. This book will help you define, find, fix, and feed healthful foods to your families. It covers the benefits and issues surrounding each food group and describes ways to shift these foods into your diet gradually. It is designed for families committed to moving toward more wholesome foods and more healthful lives.

How to Use This Book

The *Introduction* helps you to define and find nutritious foods. After exploring the difficulties associated with healthful eating, a simple guiding principle is introduced as well as the concept of "shifting." Various ways to shop for healthful foods are provided along with a discussion of organic products.

The *Real Foods* chapter is the core of this book. It reviews Basic Nutritional Information then discusses each plant (whole grains, fruits and vegetables, nuts and seeds, legumes and sweeteners) and animal (fish, poultry and eggs, dairy, and meat) food group in detail. The benefits and issues surrounding each group are examined as well as ways to shift these foods into everyday life. Each food section has clear, concise text and summary tables. The tables provide quick access to core information quickly and easily.

The *Feeding the Family* section explores the question: how do you get children to want to eat healthily? It discusses concepts pertaining to children and eating, tools for encouraging healthful eating habits, and avoiding food battles. "Safety," "Equipment," and "Age Appropriate Activities" provide detailed information about how to interest children in nutritious foods.

The *Quick Ideas and Basic Recipes* chapter includes 50 suggestions for nutritious and delicious foods. It provides a sample of the wide range of possible snacks and meals which can be made with nutrient-dense whole foods. *Quick Ideas* are short reminders about quick and easy dishes. These are explained in a few sentences and do not require a recipe. They are followed by *Basic Recipes,* which focus on simple cooking techniques. Once learned, these recipes can be easily modified for a variety of meals.

The Appendix includes a Favorite Foods List, Resources, Recommended Reading, Bibliography, and Index.

We are all chemically different, have diverse family backgrounds, and feel better eating a particular diet. We need to be aware of our bodies and family history and to work closely with our healthcare professionals to find a way of eating that is best for us. If your healthcare provider does not have a background in nutrition, try to find one who does. (See Appendix C for more information.)

Introduction

"It is ironic that in this day and time we are so over-weight, yet so malnourished."
Ann Louise Gittleman, Ph.D.

Unhealthful Eating

The "P" Generation

Many adults today are from the "P" generation. We have grown up with processed, prepared, and packaged foods. Someone else gathers, prepares, packages, and presents the food frozen, boxed, bagged, canned, or somehow sealed. We open, microwave, eat. We don't know where it came from or how, but placing it in the microwave and on the table seems easier and safer than doing any more ourselves. As a result, we are no longer connected to real food.

A recent national food survey revealed this generation is "lost in the kitchen." Ninety percent of adults between 25 and 54 considered themselves "good to excellent cooks" but 75 percent failed a basic cooking test. So many of us lack knowledge of real foods and experience in the kitchen. For me, cooking required a recipe, and a single missing ingredient meant it was time for take-out. I couldn't even identify real foods, much less cook them. If I found hulled barley or Swiss chard, I didn't know what to do with it. Talk about starting from scratch. Soak beans? Make stock? The only stock I knew was on Wall Street.

Our grandmothers cooked. They had no choice. The latest, greatest, time-saving, preservative-laden, advanced technology was not available. They had real foods and had to learn how to cook them. Our mothers probably learned to cook too, but we have been lulled by easy food: drive-throughs, vending machines, and food that keeps forever.

Easy Food

Refined, processed food is easy: easy to find, easy to make, and easy to eat. It is available practically everywhere, it's inexpensive, the instructions are on the box, and it tastes good. Companies spend millions of dollars trying to obtain the most desirable balance of salt, sweeteners, or the latest synthetic flavor from the high-tech flavoring industry. Then they make it look nice and pretty with artificial colors and provide a long shelf life by removing all those pesky, perishable nutrients. But is lengthening its life worth shortening ours?

Refined, processed foods have little or no nutrients left. In fact, they have negative nutrients. These products are not just "empty calories," they are "negative calories." When consumed, they pull nutrients from the body's own meager reserves to aid digestion. They may also tax the system with other harmful, unnatural, and unrecognizable substances. These technological "advances" have ruined the quality of our food and the quality of our health. The shortcuts and mass production may have given us cheaper food, but not better food. Just easier food without nutrients. We are disconnecting ourselves from real food at a huge cost—our health.

Conflicting and Overwhelming Information

For those trying to improve their diets, simply defining nutritious food can be a manic experience. We swerve back and forth in the grocery stores trying to decide—low-fat? Sugar-free? No cholesterol? Nutrition books offer various opinions: high protein, vegetarian, don't eat eggs, eat more eggs, butter is bad, butter is good. Everyone has their own slant, angle, or "latest research." If we close our eyes, cover our ears, and walk around humming "Na-na-na-na," doing what we have always done—eating easy, available, unhealthful food—experts will soon change their minds anyway.

Then there are the diet books with their six-week programs, formulas, and guilt for succumbing to "not-allowed" edibles. We go on a diet, off a diet, up and down, around and around, and never get anywhere. We usually end up back with our old eating habits. If it won't last, why bother?

Most cookbooks are simply recipes. They lack background nutritional information about the ingredients. They do not explain which fish are most likely to be contaminated with mercury, which sweeteners contain the most nutrients, or which oils are most appropriate for cooking. They are written by gourmets who have grown up loving to cook. Food is their life. If we want to eat healthily, we have to change our lives. But if we removed processed, refined foods from our diets, we would eliminate more than ninety percent of the food in the grocery store and fast-food restaurants. What would we eat?

More Healthful Eating

It can be challenging to shift to more nutritious foods with limited time, knowledge, money, ability, and prejudiced taste buds. As with any important change, learning to eat better requires effort and persistence but can be accomplished gradually and permanently.

Defining

Healthful eating means consuming nutrient-dense foods. The most nutrient-dense foods are whole foods*—foods in their original form; plant foods in their natural state, and animal products from animals in their natural environments, eating their natural diets. It has always made sense and will always make sense: *eat real foods.*

This principle is used to evaluate each individual food group and the issues surrounding them. It helps us explore how to obtain the maximum benefit from these foods and how to avoid damaging, depleting, or destroying the nutrients. It is a guide to interpreting the latest research, fads, and food issues. It does not change and is the one I come back to time after time.

> **Many people equate the term "whole foods" with plant-based foods and vegetarian diets. For the purpose of this book, the terms "whole foods" and "real foods" are synonymous. They are defined as all foods, plant and animal, traced back their to their natural environments and original forms.*

Shifting

Once you have defined the most healthful foods, brainstorm all the possible ways to incorporate these foods into your diet. Choose the easiest steps first and begin making changes, or "shifting." Shifting is consciously repeating actions until they become an unconscious routine, or habit. Then shift more. Find nutritious foods, eat them, and then find more. Learn basic recipes, practice them, and then learn more.

Transitioning to more healthful foods does not have to be fast or strict, but it needs to become a habit—a way of life. Take slow, small steps which evolve into permanent changes in your eating habits. The key is shifting—making gradual, but permanent changes* without shocking yourself or your family. Children, especially, do not need counting, formulas, or guilt. They need nutrients and real, healthful food.

Change can be difficult. The goal is to move from "first-order change" to "second-order" change. First-order change is a variation in the procedures within a given system, leaving the system itself relatively unchanged. Second-order change occurs when the system itself is changed. "First-order change is superficial and brief," states author and therapist Robert J. MacKenzie, Ed.D. "When the change is discontinued, old patterns of behavior return." But to move beyond the superficial change to second-order change is to develop a new system, a new pattern, a new way of eating.

Keep looking for more nutritious versions and substituting with more healthful, whole foods. Every step, every small change, every permanent shift helps. When they become habits, make more, slowly and steadily, constantly resisting the temptation to go backward. Focus on shifting, learning, enjoying, and making changes that will last.

Tools for Shifting

If you find nutritious foods and fix them well, you can truly enjoy how they taste and how they make you feel. Eating is a way of life, something you do every day, several times a day. Every time you eat is an opportunity to put nutritious food in your body. The following strategies will help you shift to more nutritious foods.

Readiness: Decide which steps you are ready for now and which ones to try later. Some changes will seem easy to you. Others will seem more difficult. Some will be more important than others. You may find that you follow some of the suggestions already. Pick and choose what works for you and your family. As you go through this book, look for ways to make the meals and snacks that you already eat more healthful. Look for new meals and snacks. Pick the easiest changes first; make a list of steps to take later. Make the switches that you are comfortable with now and maintain momentum. Keep shifting in the right direction and including more real foods in your diet.

Decisions: Decide where you can make the most impact without getting overwhelmed. For example, making soup helped me include many traditionally difficult whole foods: whole grains, vegetables, and legumes. Canned soup is not as nutritious as homemade, so it is worthwhile to make it. However, making my own broth ("stock"), at this point in my life, is unrealistic and overwhelming. So I buy it. Find the balance between maximizing nutrients from real foods and overwhelming yourself with tasks that are too complicated and may cause you to give up. Decide where to draw the line between everything made from scratch and everything processed, prepared, and packaged. Each family has to decide what changes they can handle and what needs to wait.

Attitude: Healthful eating is not about doing everything perfectly. It is a process of changing what you eat to more nutritious foods. Many people have come to equate the term "diet" with a special plan for losing weight. While weight-loss can be beneficial, the whole notion of "dieting" has done people a disservice. They focus on a special diet plan, denying themselves food rather than shifting to more healthful choices. The "plan" does not become a person's habit, and often dieters swing from one extreme or another. In reality every small change you make has impact if you maintain it.

Many people have health issues as a result of a lifetime of poor eating and now need to manage their eating in special ways. Weight maintenance is important, and a pleasant side effect of eating healthful foods, but the focus should be on consuming nutrient-dense foods as a way of life. If children grow up consuming real foods today, they will not suffer as many health consequences in the future.

Rituals: Eating is a very personal activity. People have emotional connections to particular meals and foods. Some people crave special comfort foods for breakfast or look forward to starting the day in a particular way. Others want to serve warm breads or cookies to their kids when they come home from school because of their own fond memories. There's no need to deprive yourself or give up traditions; simply try to move in a more healthful direction. Just as getting 80 percent of the way up the mountain is better than not climbing the mountain at all, improving 80 percent or even 50 percent of what we eat is a giant leap in terms of good health.

Expectations: Try to be open-minded about switching to real foods. They may look, smell, and taste different. It can be a shock to see dark, shriveled, dried fruit, peanut butter with oil floating on top, and cloudy oils and juices. But processed dried fruit looks moist and colorful because it has been treated with the preservative sulfur dioxide. The "clouds" in healthy oils and juices contain nutrients, and I would rather the oil separate from my peanut butter than have the manufacturer mix in unhealthy hydrogenated oil to make it look smooth. Beware of pretty packages and get used to food in its natural form, rich with flavors, smells, textures, and nutrients. Besides, what is really important—how something looks or the quality of what is inside?

Keep educating yourself, set goals, and stay motivated. Find other like-minded people. What do they eat? How do they feed their families? Share ideas, recipes, books, tips, strategies, and don't be afraid to ask silly questions. Every little bit counts. Feel good about what you do for yourself and your family.

The Organic Question

To shift to a real foods diet, do you have to eat organic foods? No. To obtain the most nutritious foods possible, do you have to eat organic? Probably. When I first began making changes in my diet, it was difficult including vegetables at all. If I had to buy organic food as well, I would have given up right then. Eating whole foods can be challenging enough. But in my quest for the most nutritious foods, I eventually came to a point when I was ready to explore "the organic question." Not only are organic foods more nutrient dense, they contain the least amount of harmful substances.* If you truly want the most healthful foods, make an extra effort to include organic.

While studies have demonstrated organic foods contain more nutrients and fewer toxins, there are variations. Locally grown conventional produce picked at its peak is probably a better choice than overripe, bruised organic produce. Many grass-fed meat products contain more nutrients but do not meet all of the standards required by the National Organic Program. However, farmers and ranchers conscious enough to pasture-raise animals probably follow the organic model closely and produce quality products.

---

1. **Organic products contain more nutrients.** Organic farmers work with nature. Their soil is rich with nutrients from composting and rotating crops. The soil from "industrialized agriculture" has been depleted of nutrients, needing supplemental chemicals and synthetic fertilizers.

2. **Organic products contain fewer toxins.** Toxins can lead to neurological and other health–related problems. Pesticides, herbicides, and fungicides are toxins designed to kill. I realize I am a larger organism than the ones these poisons target, but I also consume a large amount of food over a long period of time with many different food (and pesticide) combinations. The developing systems of babies and children are more susceptible to toxins, and they eat proportionally

more food because of their rapid growth.

3. Agricultural chemicals harm the environment. Pesticides also kill the beneficial organisms which help keep the soil healthy and fertile. Many are persistent. Designed to endure the elements: heat, cold, water, and time, they remain on the food or in the air, soil, rivers, lakes, oceans, and other living organisms.

4. Buying organic food is an investment. Buying organic is usually more expensive. I view it as an investment in my health and the health of my family. I am saving money on medications we won't need and doctors' bills we won't have in the future because we are healthier. It is also my small contribution toward a better, cleaner, healthier world for future generations.

Eating whole foods, organic or not, is what's important. Do not use lack of organic products as an excuse to eat refined. In fact, refined organic products are now a growing market. It is better to eat a conventional (non-organic) apple than refined, organic cookies. Any step away from refined products to real foods is an enormous accomplishment. Organic products are simply one more step in the process of shifting to more healthful, more nutritious foods.

Do not to agonize over this issue either. Try to be as informed as possible, make educated decisions about the foods you eat, and trust your body's natural mechanisms to rid itself of toxins. Some organic products are more important than others. Key issues are discussed in their respective food sections and further resources can be found in Appendix C.

Make an effort to find organic whole food products. They are the most healthful, most nutritious foods available. If life gets too hectic, choose natural, whole foods. It's a balancing act: prioritize, find ways to make life easier (freezing foods, buying in bulk, etc.), and let go when life gets crazy. Suggestions for finding organic products are described in the next section.

*The USDA National Organic Program implemented new labeling standards in October 2002 stating that organic products are grown without the use of toxic, persistent pesticides and fertilizers, and prohibit the use of genetic engineering, irradiation, sewage sludge, growth hormones, and antibiotics. All products labeled "organic" must now meet these standards.

Shopping and Buying

Take a moment to review where and how you obtain the foods you eat. Do you shop once a week at the supermarket? Make frequent stops at convenience stores or fast-food restaurants? Research and evaluate the other resources in your area. Is there a small health food store nearby? Where is the nearest natural foods supermarket? What about farmstands, farmers' markets, and community farms? Is there a fish market, food cooperative or buying club? Each of these choices are explained below.

Supermarkets: It is possible to shift to a diet of real foods and continue shopping at the regular supermarket. You may be avoiding about 90 percent of the products in the store, but the remaining 10 percent will provide a balanced diet of real foods. Try to plan before shopping and make sure each food group is represented. Start by taking a new look at your regular grocery store. Shop the periphery. Most real foods are found on the outer aisles.

Spend time in the produce department and choose from different food families: berries, citrus, greens, root vegetables, squashes, etc. If peeled and cut produce increases the likelihood of its being eaten, buy it. It will, however, spoil more quickly. Purchase new foods as well as familiar favorites, but plan well. It can be frustrating to waste quality food and money on unused perishable produce. Become familiar with the Environmental Working Group's "Shopper's Guide to Pesticides in Produce" (p.42) and choose accordingly. If organic products are unavailable, buy from the "least contaminated" list, local produce in season, or frozen organic.

Next, buy grains and beans. Look for sealed packages with cooking instructions and recipes. Canned beans, tomato products, and other canned produce are also options. Check the "international" food aisle for a wider selection. (I purchase nuts and seeds at the health food store—organic and refrigerated, if possible.)

Finally, look for cold food items: dairy, meats, fish, poultry, and eggs. Is there a quality meat and seafood department? Do they carry organic dairy products? Grass-fed meats? Is there a "natural foods" section? Toxins tend to settle in fats, so organic is a more healthful choice for nuts, seeds, oils, dairy, meat and other products containing fat. Organic dairy, meat, poultry, and eggs are free of growth hormones and antibiotics and are becoming more popular in regular grocery stores. Find products you like and develop new shopping habits until these become routine. If you discover holes in your diet or need more variety, find the nearest health food store.

Health Food Stores: These can range from small stores with a sampling of natural and organic products to large natural foods supermarkets such as Whole Foods Markets and Wild Oats. They offer more variety and, often, better-quality natural and organic food products. Check the phonebook under "health food store" and "natural food store," or search the Internet. If you have a distance to travel, consider bringing a cooler for refrigerated and frozen food items. Start looking around, reading labels, and finding products you like. Plan for perishables. It is tempting to stock up on quality, fresh foods, especially if you have traveled, but be realistic about what you have time to prepare and eat.

The advantage of shopping at a separate health food store is the wide variety of wholesome products, but don't be fooled. The term "organic" has become a popular marketing tool. It is still important to read labels. "Evaporated cane juice" is sugar cane juice. Organic sugar is still sugar, and organic white flour is still refined. Buying organic cookies, cakes, cereals, crackers, and snacks can be a step in the right direction, but don't stop there. There are more healthful, more nutritious choices. Keep moving.

Local Farms: Local farmstands, farmers' markets, and community sustainable agriculture (CSA) are also options. They carry produce picked at its peak, full of flavor and nutrients, and often organic. If you want to know more, ask the farmers. They tend to use fewer pesticides and can even offer cooking suggestions. CSAs are small farms supported by community members who buy "shares" to help pay for the operating budget. In return, they receive a share of the harvest (usually organic). These local farms are spreading across the nation. Find out if there is one near you. Fresh-picked, organic produce—what could be better? Growing your own vegetables is another option but may not be realistic for many busy families.

Food Cooperatives and Buying Clubs: These are groups of local people who come together to order natural and organic foods in bulk. Buying products wholesale can save time, money, and bring together health-minded individuals. Online and mail-order resources are also available, but shipping adds an extra expense (see Appendix B).

I begin the month buying in bulk from our food cooperative catalog. I often split cases with friends and find new foods we love to eat. Then I travel to a large natural foods supermarket with my coolers to stock up. I purchased an upright freezer for the basement to store cases of frozen food from the buying club and extra from the health food store. Throughout the month I supplement with produce from local farms, fresh fish from the fish market, items from the local grocery store or smaller health food store, and, during the growing season, produce from a community farm and our own small garden. The better I plan, the less shopping I do.

In the *Real Foods* section, I have tried to explain the transition to whole, nutrient-dense foods in a clear and simple manner. Suggestions for obtaining the highest-quality nutrients are organized from the easiest to the most difficult. Some of these concepts may seem unrealistic, overwhelming, and to go against conventional advice. As you read, try to be open and trust your own instincts. You do not have to make all of these changes at once, or at all for that matter, but you never know what opportunities may present themselves down the road.

Happy reading and healthful eating.

Real Foods

Basic Nutritional Information

Macronutrients: Proteins, Fats, and Carbohydrates

The body requires three types of nutrients to function properly: macronutrients, micronutrients, and water. Macronutrients (proteins, fats, and carbohydrates) provide energy and help maintain and repair the body, and are needed in larger amounts than micronutrients.

Protein is essential for growth, maintenance and repair. It is the primary structural material of the body and is needed for the manufacture of hormones, antibodies, enzymes, and tissues. Proteins are composed of "building blocks" called amino acids which are broken are used by the body. There are two kinds of amino acids: essential, which must be obtained from the diet, and nonessential, which can be made by the body. Proteins from animal sources such as meat, fish, eggs, and dairy contain all the essential amino acids and are considered "complete." The protein found in most grains, legumes (beans, peanuts, and peas), and leafy green vegetables are incomplete (except soybeans) and need to be paired with other complementary protein sources to provide all of the essential amino acids. Combining grains with legumes or nuts and seeds forms a complete protein.

Fats are essential for energy, brain development, hormone production, immune function, and other metabolic activities. Fats are made up of building blocks called fatty acids. There are three major types of naturally occurring fats—saturated, monounsaturated, and polyunsaturated. Saturated fatty acids are found primarily in animal products; monounsaturated in plant and nut oils such as olive, sunflower, and canola; and polyunsaturated in plant oils like flax, safflower, and walnut and include essential fatty acids. Essential fatty acids (EFAs) are vital in promoting overall health and must be obtained from the diet.

Carbohydrates supply the body with energy and are found mostly in plant foods. They are divided into two groups: simple and complex. Simple carbohydrates, sometimes called simple sugars, include fructose (fruit sugar), sucrose (table sugar), and lactose (milk sugar), as well as other sugars. Fruits are one of the richest natural sources of simple carbohydrates. Complex carbohydrates are also made up of sugars but form a longer, more complex chain. They are found in whole grains, vegetables, and legumes. Carbohydrates, except for undigested fiber, are converted to glucose and provide energy for the cells. The fiber provides further health benefits by helping to cleanse the digestive tract and lower excess cholesterol.

Micronutrients: Vitamins, Minerals, and Phytonutrients

Micronutrients (vitamins and minerals), needed in smaller amounts, are also essential for the body to function and help maintain normal metabolism. They are found in abundance in whole grains, fruits, vegetables, legumes, nuts, and seeds. These foods also contain important phytonutrients which help protect the body and fight disease.

Phytonutrients are protective, disease-fighting compounds found in plants. Often referred to as phytochemicals, they are not "essential" for life but can optimize health with their antioxidant, anti-cancer, and heart-protecting substances. Hundreds of phytonutrients have already been identified and hundreds more have yet to be discovered. They fall into categories such as carotenoids, flavonoids, indoles, and phenols.

Plant Foods

"Since the advent of chemical and industrial methods of agriculture, however, the soil in our major growing areas has been treated like dirt." Chris Kilham, *The Whole Food Bible*

Plants need water, sun, and soil to grow. The most nutrient-dense plant foods have access to fertile soil, a clean environment, and are picked at their peak. This ideal, however, can become compromised in various ways.

Modern agricultural methods often farm one type of crop repeatedly (monoculture), depleting the soil of nutrients. The use of insecticides, fungicides, and other agricultural chemicals destroy important living compounds such as insects, earthworms, and bacteria which help maintain soil health. Without them, soil becomes sterile and dies. Farmers become trapped in a continuous cycle of needing chemical fertilizers to keep their land productive.

An increasing number of plants are genetically engineered to grow bigger, faster, or stronger. They are harvested prematurely to travel long distances and may be treated with artificial preservation techniques or stored improperly, further depleting nutrients.

Farmers are burdened with hefty chemicals bills, the once-fertile land is eroding, blowing, or washing away, and we are left with persistent chemicals in our environment. This is a high price to pay—for the farmers, the environment, and our health. It is also unnecessary.

Sustainable agricultural methods produce nutrient-dense foods farmed in fertile soil from composting, crop rotation, and nutrient-rich ground covers which are turned back into the ground. The soil is alive with organic matter and beneficial organisms. Naturally strong plants ward off pests and problems or are helped by farmers using natural management techniques so as not to harm our food, environment, or health. Nutrient-dense foods are picked at their peak and fresh for the table. Get real.

REFINED→ → → → → → → → → → → → → → → → → → →REAL		
Nutrients depleted, removed, destroyed, or rendered harmful	Closer to original form	Whole
	Less processed	Nutrient-dense
Additives: artificial colors, flavors, or sweeteners, binders, bleaching agents, chemical leaveners, conditioners, emulsifiers, fat substitutes, fillers, preservatives, synthetic nutrients	Fewer toxins	Original form
	More whole	Natural state
	More nutrients	Clean
		Safe
		Nutritious
Processing		
Removing		
Extracting		
Exposing		
Filtering		
Clarifying		
Deodorizing		
Coloring		

GRAINS	Bleached flour Treated with dough conditioners Preservatives Synthetically enriched Bread products with additives	Unbleached refined flour High-heat milling Grains with bran and germ removed	Cracked grains Steel-cut oats Rolled grains Stone-ground, whole grain flours	Whole grains
PRODUCE	Dried fruits with sulfur dioxide Canned produce with syrups and additives	Canned produce Frozen produce	Fresh	Local, organic fruits and vegetables
NUTS /SEEDS	Partially hydro-genated and hydro-genated oils	High-heat processing Solvent extracted Refined Deodorized Clarified	Ground nut butters Expeller-pressed oil Unrefined	Whole nuts and seeds
LEGUMES	Refined soy products (soy protein isolate, oil, flour)	Canned beans with additives	Unrefined, fermented soy products Canned beans	Dried beans, peas, and lentils
SWEETENERS	High fructose corn syrup Corn syrup Syrups with additives Sugar alcohols (isomalt, maltitol, mannitol) Artificial sweeteners	White sugar Brown sugar Refined molasses Jams with additives Sugar alcohols (xylitol, sorbitol)	Grain syrups Raw sugar Natural jams	Natural sweeteners Honey Pure maple syrup Unrefined molasses Stevia (sweet herb)

Table 1 : Plant Foods

Whole Grains

*"Consumption of sugar and white flour may be likened to drawing
on a savings account. If continued withdrawals are made faster
than new funds are put in, the account will eventually become
depleted."* —Sally Fallon, *Nourishing Traditions*

Is there a difference between "wheat bread" and "whole-wheat
bread?" Does it matter what type of rice you buy? What about oatmeal?
If grains are ground to make flour, how can you have "whole grain"
flour? Learning about whole grains can be confusing, and they can be
hard to find. Some products are not sold in regular supermarkets. Health
food stores can be intimidating enough with their bins and bags of unfamiliar foods and aisles of vitamins and supplements, not to mention
unpronounceable products such as quinoa (keen'wa) and amaranth.
Following the real foods guiding principle will help you find the most
nutritious products.

Benefits: Grains are the seeds and fruits of cereal grasses. We
consume products made mostly with some form of wheat (hard, soft,
winter, spring, or durum), but there are also barley, oats, rice, and other
less popular grains such as amaranth, buckwheat, millet, and quinoa. In
their natural, whole-grain state, they are a valuable source of complex
carbohydrates, proteins, unsaturated fats, B vitamins, vitamin E, iron,
zinc, magnesium, fiber, and other vitamins and minerals. These grains
can be soaked, sprouted, cooked whole, cracked, rolled (flaked), or
ground into flours. Cracked and rolled grains are often used for cereals
and ground grains (flour) for breads and pasta.

Issues: The main issues surrounding grains are refining and the
use of undesirable additives. Grains consist of three layers: the germ,
bran, and endosperm. When grains are refined, the high-fiber, outer
layer of bran and the nutrient-dense, perishable germ are removed.

The remaining endosperm is ground into flour, using high-speed roller milling. The heat created can damage or destroy nutrients. The flour is further processed with artificial bleaching and maturing agents which take minutes instead of months, rather than allowing the flour to mature naturally during storage.

Flour is combined with a leavener, water, and other ingredients to make bread and various bread products. Some manufacturers use questionable additives such as emulsifiers, accelerators, and other dough conditioners and preservatives to enhance taste, texture, and appearance. Finally, after most of the nutrients have been depleted, removed, or destroyed, and a handful of synthetic nutrients (usually thiamin, niacin, riboflavin, and iron) added, the product is then labeled "enriched" or "fortified."

Refined grain products such as white rice, white bread, and processed cereals made from refined flour supply the body with energy but little else. In fact, consuming products made with refined flour (and sugar) actually depletes the body's own storehouse of nutrients. The missing nutrients must be pulled from bones, tissues, and other reserves in order to metabolize the nutrient-lacking, refined product. They have little, no, or negative nutrient value, are laden with unnecessary and undesirable additives, can cause dramatic fluctuations of blood sugar levels, and are high glycemic foods.

The glycemic index (GI) measures how quickly a carbohydrate is digested and raises blood sugar levels. Carbohydrates are consumed, measured, and ranked according to their immediate effect on blood glucose (blood sugar) levels. Pure glucose (sugar) and white bread have a relatively high score of 100 on the glycemic index. (Low GI foods are less than 55; high GI foods are greater than 70.) Now researchers are measuring the glycemic *load* (GL) of foods to provide a more accurate picture of the impact on body chemistry. (Low GL foods are less than 10; high GL foods are greater than 20.) The glycemic load is calculated by multiplying the glycemic index by the amount of carbohydrate in the food. For example, raw carrots have a high glycemic index of 131, but they contain only 4 grams of carbohydrate, for a low glycemic load of 5 (131% x 4).

Processed, refined white flour products are typically high glycemic foods. They are rapidly digested and absorbed, causing a quick rise in blood sugar levels, energy, and insulin. Insulin is produced by the pancreas to manage sugar. When the sugar is used quickly, the excess insulin leads to cravings for more, and an addictive cycle is created. During the short term, this causes dramatic effects on energy levels, moods swings, and attention span. Over time, the insulin response begins to wear out and possibly lead to weight gain, diabetes, heart disease, and cancer. It is most desirable to consume whole grains and whole-grain products. They digest slowly, providing a steady supply of energy as well as other nutrients and fiber. (For more information see table p.29 or Appendix B.)

Unrefined, whole grains can be soaked, sprouted, cooked, cracked, rolled, or ground. They can be combined with other real, quality ingredients to make nutritious, healthful products. Millers grind whole grain flours using slow, low-temperature, stone-grinding or hammer-milling to protect delicate nutrients from damage. Even if the bran and germ are removed, refined wheat flour can mature naturally in storage rather than being treated with bleaching and maturing agents. Real food ingredients can be added to enhance the flavor, texture, appearance, and to preserve products naturally. Read labels. If the list of additives is long and unfamiliar, find something else to eat.

We have two choices: learn about and consume nutritious whole grains and whole-grain products or choose foods from manufacturers who strip the grains of close to 30 nutrients, refine them into a starchy, bleached powder laden with additives, then add back a few synthetic vitamins and call them "enriched." As author and nutritionist Robert Crayhon said, "If someone took $30,000 from you and then gave you $4,000, would you feel enriched?"

Shifting: Without the perishable nutrients, refined flour has a long shelf life and is a popular choice with manufacturers. It seems to be everywhere and in everything: bread products, cookies, crackers, cereal, mixes, chips, and many other snack foods. On the other hand, the nutrients in whole-grain products diminish over time. So select whole-grain versions you know you will use and change the type of snacks and meals you serve to fruits, nuts, dairy, and other foods. Also limit refined products to when you have specific goals in mind. For example, consuming vegetables mixed with a favorite refined pasta or beans in a white flour tortilla are understandable compromises if eating vegetables or beans is the priority.

If you use white rice, change to brown; replace instant oatmeal with rolled oats; and buy small bags of stone-ground whole-wheat flour to increasingly mix with unbleached white for baking. For every cup of white flour used, replace ¼ cup with whole-wheat flour. This will ease the transition on your taste buds. Read the labels of the grain products you normally buy (pasta, cereals, and bread items) and look for "whole grains" or "whole-grain flours" in the ingredients. "Wheat flour" is refined, so look for the word "whole." Also look for natural, real food ingredients and additives. Since the natural oils in whole-grain flour can become rancid, use fresh products quickly and store them properly.

Next, become familiar with the whole grains available in your supermarket. Look for prepackaged, sealed bags with cooking instructions and recipes. Also check the "natural foods" or "international foods" sections. Use quick-cooking grains (rice, quinoa, or buckwheat) for dinner or get into the habit of having precooked grains on hand in the refrigerator for soups, salads, or side dishes. Longer-cooking grains (barley, oat groats, or wheat berries) can simmer while you eat. They will be done as you finish and ready for the next day. Or cook them in the morning and use half for a salad at lunch and the rest at dinner. Mix rice with beans, vegetables, and vinaigrette dressing for a salad, put extra barley in a soup, or sauté vegetables and add other cooked grains for a pilaf-type side dish. If you like oatmeal for breakfast, try steel-cut oats, millet, and other multi-grain hot cereals. Experiment with other whole grain flours. Pair grains with beans for at least one meal a week. They contain different types of proteins and complement each other well.

Finally, make a trip to a health food store for more variety and better-quality whole-grain products. Buy grains in bulk to cut down on costs and look for organic products. To receive the maximum benefit from whole grains, toast, soak, sprout, and even grind them at home. Toasting grains can add flavor and reduce cooking time. Soaking grains overnight, or a few hours before cooking, decreases cooking time, aids digestion, and increases nutrient absorption by breaking down phytic acid, a substance in seeds which can inhibit the absorption of minerals.

Try using a rice cooker, slow cooker, pressure cooker, or soak grains during the night and cook them in the morning while exercising or showering. Then enjoy them throughout the day as a warm breakfast porridge, on a salad for lunch, and as a side dish or even the base of a main meal, with beans, for dinner.

Sprouted grains are also nutritious and easy to digest. Look for sprouted-grain bread products in the freezer section of health food stores. Another option is to order fresh, stone-milled flours by mail (see Appendix B) or grind your own (see *Equipment* in Appendix C.) There are hand and electric grinders, and some blenders and food processors also will grind grains (check the manuals).

Some people have food sensitivities or allergies to grains. Gluten, the protein found in many grains, provides the elastic qualities which help hold breads and pasta together. It can also be difficult to digest. Gluten-free grains and alternative food sources are available for those who want to remove glutens from their diet (see Appendix B). Others may feel better limiting, managing, or removing grains to help maintain blood sugar levels.

Storing: Store whole grains in tightly sealed containers up to six months in the pantry or up to one year in the refrigerator, especially during hot, humid weather. Sealed glass or sturdy, plastic containers are best. Mason jars or old pasta sauce containers work well. Bags may encourage bugs. Cooked grains can be stored in the refrigerator for two to three days or frozen. Having pre-cooked grains on hand for a soup, salad, or side dish can be a helpful time saver.

Store ground grains in their original bags, encased in another zipper-lock type bag, in the refrigerator or freezer. Grinding exposes the fats in grains to oxygen, causing them to oxidize, or spoil. Unbleached, refined flour can be stored in the pantry. Use whole-grain bread products within a few days or freeze them.

My family purchased an extra upright freezer for our basement for added storage space. Compared to chest freezers, upright freezers make it easier to see what you have and to rotate food. The more whole or intact the grain, the longer it will take to cook. So plan ahead and cook extra for leftovers.

Shifting Summary

Start with:

- *brown rice, rolled oats, and more "whole"-some grain products*
- *unbleached white flour for baking; replace one quarter to one-third with whole-wheat flour*
- *whole grains and whole-grain products available in regular supermarkets*

Shift to:

- *steel-cut oats or other multi-grain hot cereals; other whole-grain flours*
- *pre-cook whole grains (barley, buckwheat, or quinoa); add to a soup, salad, pilaf, or as a side dish*
- *sprouted-grain bread products; pairing grains and beans at meals*

Most nutritious:

- *Visit health food stores for (organic) whole grains and whole-grain flours*
- *Consider soaking, sprouting, and grinding your own grains*
- *Research natural food cooperatives, buying clubs, and mail-order grain products*

MANAGING THE GLYCEMIC IMPACT OF FOODS*

Factors Influencing the Glycemic Impact of Foods:

Processing: grinding, refining, and "swelling" foods can increase the
surface area, rate of digestion, and, in turn, their glycemic value
(popped corn, instant oatmeal, and puffed rice cakes)

Fiber: the intact fibrous coating (whole grains and legumes) and soluble
fibers (rolled oats and apples) slow digestion and lower glycemic values

Type of Starch and Sugar: certain types of starch (amylose found in most
legumes and some types of rice) and sugar (the fructose found in apple
and oranges) tend to have lower glycemic values (fruit juices, however,
with more sugar and less fiber, have higher glycemic values)

Whole Foods: unrefined foods also contribute other valuable nutrients
(vitamins, minerals, fiber, and phytonutrients)

High Glycemic Foods	Medium Glycemic Foods	Low Glycemic Foods
White-flour products	Starchy vegetables	Vegetables
Processed-grain products	Bananas	Legumes
Potatoes, mashed	Pineapples	Dairy
Soft drinks	Fruit juices	Fruits (berries)
Candy	Honey	Whole grains

*Rather than memorizing glycemic tables, become familiar with the
system and the types of foods in each category. Use it as a tool or strategy
to make more informed food choices.

**Individuals can have different reactions or "sensitivities" to particular
foods. Some may feel a quick surge of energy followed by a rapid drop
after eating a baked potato; others may find potatoes supply a steady
source of energy. Use your discoveries as a means to help make the best
choices. (See Appendix B for more information.)

Table 2 : Managing the Glycemic Impact of Foods

WHOLE GRAINS

What to Limit or Eliminate:
Refined grains; products with unnecessary or undesirable additives
Spoiled whole grains: grains need to be kept away from air, light, and
   moisture
Wheat and wheat products: a widely used grain and common allergen*

What to Add or Increase:
Whole grains: cracked, rolled, or ground (see "WHOLE-GRAIN
   FLOURS")
Whole-grain products

Whole Grain	Description and Uses
Amaranth	Small yellow seed with crunchy texture; contains protein, calcium, iron; gluten-free; use in cereals or mix with other grains in pilafs and salads
Barley	Nutty, chewy grain; hulled barley (outer fibrous layer intact) contains protein, fiber, and B-vitamins; pearled barley has outer hull removed; use in soups, salads, casseroles, and pilafs; also available in flakes and grits
Brown Rice	Available in short (chewy), medium, and long grains; contains fiber, protein, and vitamin E; use as a side or in soup, salad, pilaf, or casserole; wild rice is actually the seed of an aquatic grass
Buckwheat	Kasha (toasted buckwheat); nutritional value similar to wheat but gluten-free; contains thiamin, riboflavin, calcium, and phosphorus; use in salads and pilafs
Millet	Tiny gold seed; contains thiamin, iron, protein, potassium; easily digested, gluten-free; use in hot cereals, puddings, and soups
Oats	Available as whole oat groats, sliced or steel-cut (Scotch) oats, or rolled (steamed, flattened) oats, or quick-cooking (thinner rolled) oatmeal; high in soluble fiber, protein, and B-vitamins; use in cereals or whole oats in soups and salads
Quinoa	Small, pearly "super grain;" a complete protein with calcium, iron, phosphorus, and B-vitamins; gluten-free, use in salads and pilafs

Whole Grain	Description and Uses
Rye	Hearty, long-cooking grain (used mostly as flour); grows in poor soil, harsh climates; triticale is hybrid of wheat and rye; also available in flakes
Wheat	Available whole (wheat berries), cracked (bulgur), and precooked pasta (couscous); high in protein, B-vitamins, iron, zinc, and fiber; use in soups, salads, or pilafs; most popular grain in North America, mostly for flour and baked goods
Tips: Soak grains overnight to maximize nutrient absorption, aid digestion, and shorten cooking time Add a bay leaf wrapped in cheese cloth (to avoid sharp edges) or mint tea bag to containers to discourage bugs	
How to Store: It is best to refrigerate (mason jars work well) or freeze grains in closed containers for four to five months, especially in a hot, humid climate (or store in a cool, dry place) Refrigerate cooked grains three to four days or freeze	

Table 3 : Whole Grains

*Gluten is a protein found in wheat and other grains (barley, rye, oat, kamut, triticale, and spelt). Some people have difficulty digesting gluten and may want to seek other grain sources. (See Appendix B for more information.)

WHOLE-GRAIN FLOURS

What to Limit or Eliminate:

Refined flours (germ and bran removed): white, wheat, or enriched flour

Bleached flour treated with dough conditioners, preservatives, and synthetic nutrients

Flours milled at high temperatures (heat from high-speed milling destroys nutrients)

Pasta and bread products with unnecessary or undesirable additives

What to Add or Increase

Unbleached white flour

Stone-ground, whole-grain flours

Whole Grain Flour	Description and Uses
Amaranth	High protein; nutty flavor; gluten-free, combine with other flours or binders to hold together; can be expensive
Barley	Sweet, malty flavor
Buckwheat	Dark, heavy; combine with other flours or binders to hold together; gluten free
Cornmeal	Use whole yellow or whole white; "bolted" has fiber removed
Millet	Sweet flavor; use quickly or store in freezer; combine with other flours or binders to hold together
Oat	Sweet flavor; combine with other flours; grind fresh from rolled oats
Rice	Gluten-free; combine with other flours or binders
Rye	Heavy texture; combine with other flours; also triticale flour (hybrid of wheat and rye)
Spelt	Popular wheat relative; readily absorbs, reduces liquid content up to 25%
Wheat	High gluten content responsible for elastic qualities in bread dough; varieties include hard, soft (pastry flour for lighter baked goods), and durum used for pasta (semolina is refined durum)

Tips:
Mix whole-grain flours with unbleached white for baking: start by replacing one-quarter unbleached white with whole-grain flour then experiment with more or other varieties
Use xatham gum to help hold gluten-free flours together
Make bread crumbs from stale bread by pulsing in food processor
How to Store:
Refrigerate small amounts in original bags, tightly sealed, for one to two months
Freeze for up to six months
If flour has a bitter taste, it has become rancid—discard

Table 4 : Whole-grain Flours

COOKING GRAINS (Stovetop)			
Directions: Rinse grains and combine with water or stock in a large pot. Bring to a boil, cover and simmer, without stirring, until water is absorbed.			
Grain (1 cup)	Liquid	Cooking Time	Yield
Amaranth	2 cups	20-25 minutes	2 cups
Barley (hulled)	3 cups	90 minutes	3 - 4 cups
Barley (pearled)	3 cups	60 minutes	3 cups
Buckwheat (ka-sha)	2 cups	15-20 minutes	3 cups
Millet	2 ½ cups	20 minutes	3 - 4 cups
Oats (whole groats)	4 cups	60 minutes	2 - 2 ½ cups
Oats (steel-cut)	3 cups	45 minutes	2 cups
Oats (rolled)	2 ½ cups	10-15 minutes	2 cups
Quinoa	2 cups	15 minutes	3 cups
Rice (brown)	2 cups	45 minutes	3 cups
Rice (basmati)	2 cups	15 minutes	3 cups
Rice (wild)	3 ½ cups	60 minutes	3 ½ cups
Rye (berries)	3 cups	90-120 minutes	2 ½ cups
Wheat berries (whole)	3 cups	60-90 minutes	2 cups
Wheat (cracked/ bulgur)	2 cups	20 minutes	3 cups
Wheat (cous-cous)	2 cups (boiling)	1 minute, remove from heat for 5 minutes, covered	3 cups
*Presoak longer-cooking grains (hulled barley, oat groats, rye, and wheat berries) to reduce cooking time. Using a pressure cooker also decreases cooking time while increasing nutrients and flavor.			

Table 5 : Cooking Grains

Vegetables and Fruits

"Eating more fruits and vegetables, in whatever form, is clearly an excellent way to improve your diet and take advantage of the healing properties of food." Andrew Weil, M.D., *Eating Well for Optimum Health*

I used to speed past the produce aisle. Fruits and vegetables always went bad before I had a chance to eat them, so I didn't buy them. Now my husband complains because the produce bin is filled with produce. Where is he supposed to put his beer? The challenge with produce is getting the right rotation of it through the house. This can be difficult during the colder months, especially if you have picky eaters and have to travel for quality food. It is tempting to stock up but frustrating when good food goes bad. Now I spend more time in the produce aisle than any other.

Benefits: Vegetables and fruits are excellent sources for carbohydrates, vitamins, minerals, fiber, and phytonutrients. Vegetables are especially nutrient dense. They are low in calories, do not contain fat or cholesterol, and generally have a low glycemic index, which helps regulate blood sugar levels.

Fruits contain natural sugars and fiber which make them a perfect snack and quick source of energy. They are also significant sources for antioxidants and phytonutrients such as vitamin C and carotenoids, which help fight disease and prevent damage to cells from chemicals called free radicals. The most nutrient-dense produce is from local, organic farmers who know how to replenish the soil and rotate crops. Produce should be picked at its peak and eaten at the height of freshness.

Issues: Avoiding pesticides and waxes, and finding quality, off-season produce can be the biggest challenges. Conventional produce, emphasizing high yields, is one of the most heavily sprayed crops. Pesticides are toxins designed to kill bugs weeds, fungi, and other "pests."

Research, testing, and debate about the safety of pesticides is an ongoing process. New information or updated testing procedures reveal chemicals previously thought safe should be banned, as happened in the past with DDT, chlordane, and dursban. Then companies introduce new products into the market and the process begins again.

The Environmental Working Group (EWG), a not-for-profit environmental research organization states, "The absence of knowledge is not proof of safety." In fact, the information about health-related issues from pesticide exposure, even at low doses, is growing. Fetuses, infants, and young children are particularly vulnerable to chemical toxins during critical stages of development.

Try to limit exposure to toxins by consuming organic produce or choosing from EWG's "Lowest in Pesticides" list (see table p 42.) Washing produce helps remove some pesticides, but many chemicals are absorbed into the fruit or vegetable. Wax and food-grade shellacs are also applied to some produce to seal in moisture and extend shelf life. This seals in toxins as well and cannot be effectively removed with washing. Peeling removes more pesticides and waxes, but also more nutrients. (For more information, visit the EWG Web site at www.ewg.org or see Appendix B. Specific information on pesticides in produce, as well as a wallet-sized Shopper's Guide card, can be found at their companion site www.foodnews.org.)

This is a difficult situation—we want the nutrients but not the chemicals. Organic can be expensive and hard to find. Sometimes conventional is all that is available. Take it one step at a time. Look for organic produce first, then supplement with conventional produce from the "Lowest in Pesticides" list. If you buy other produce or some on the "Highest in Pesticides" list, wash and peel it. Stock up on frozen organic produce, especially when cases go on sale through a food cooperative. In winter, do the best you can—wash, peel, eat, and don't worry. A healthy body will manage a few extra toxins.

Modern transportation has allowed for greater variety and availability of produce, but many foods travel more than 1,500 miles to reach your plate. Produce is often picked prematurely to avoid spoiling, never reaching its full nutrient potential. More nutrients are lost during transit.

For colder regions, however, once the growing season is over, winter can seem very sparse. Fresh produce, no matter where it came from, when, or how, can be a welcome treat.

So enjoy those late-season fruits and vegetables (apples, pears, and squashes), hunt around for fresh organic and quality conventional produce, stock up on frozen organic, and remember that canned is better than nothing. Spring will come again!

Shifting: "Eat your vegetables." The battle cry can be heard across the nation. Parents want their kids to eat them, kids know this and resist, both sides dig in, tempers flare—there has to be another way.

The first step is to brainstorm every conceivable means of getting produce, especially vegetables, into daily meals and snacks. If children are exposed to produce constantly throughout the day, it takes the pressure off eating it at one particular time. Children will see it again at the next meal, the meal after that, and so on. Buy quality, great-tasting produce, prepare it well, enjoy it yourself, make lots of "yummy" sounds, and move on.

Next, try to involve children in the planning and preparation. Give them choices of what they would like to eat. They can choose the vegetables to put in cooked eggs, what to put in soups or on a sandwich, and which vegetable to have with dinner. Have a taste-testing with produce and dips for snacks. Work with your children's hunger cycles and have produce ready when they are. (See **Feeding the Family** section or *Recommended Reading* in Appendix D for more information.)

Try having fresh vegetables and salad with dinner every night. Rotate through the different vegetable families for a variety of nutrients (roots, cruciferous, squashes, and dark leafy greens.) If possible, let children pick the vegetables at the store and for meals. Steam vegetables to preserve the nutrients, blanch (boil), or sauté in a little olive oil or butter. Quality produce should not need additional sauces or toppings, but they can be enticing additions for picky eaters. Use leftover vegetables in eggs for breakfast the next day or in a soup, stir-fry, or casserole. Include old favorites as well as new vegetables to increase variety and expand repertoires. Keep frozen vegetables, applesauce, and quality canned (without additives, organic, if possible) on hand for emergencies.

For salads, buy pre-washed, bagged, mixed greens for busy nights, another head of darker lettuce (iceberg lettuce is mostly water) for when you have time to wash and tear (a great job for kids), and finally, romaine hearts, which last longer. Be creative with enticing toppings: nuts, seeds, crumbled or shredded cheeses, and fresh or dried fruit. Put the salad in a bowl on the table and invite your family members to serve themselves. Encourage children to "try it" (which, at first, will be picking out their favorite toppings and leaving the rest—see "Toppings" p. 142) or use individual bowls so everyone can choose their own toppings.

Make the salad first so it is ready for famished children who can't wait. They will be less likely to reach for other snacks, and you won't be tempted to skip it in the hectic pre-dinner rush. Salad dressings on top or for "dipping" can provide extra encouragement, but look for quality brands made with real food ingredients. (Yes, salad dressings are "so easy to make," but if you are making numerous so-easy-to-make items, it is not so easy anymore. I keep a few from the health food store on hand.) Leftover salad becomes lunch the next day.

Then there are meals which already contain vegetables: stews, chilies, casseroles, stir-fries, pilafs, and pastas. If children love pasta, mix in a few fresh vegetables. Make Your Own Meals (MYOM) such as pizzas, burritos, and tacos. Let children choose their own ingredients. These meals make for excellent opportunities to include lots of fresh, nutritious vegetables; and everyone can choose favorites. Make vegetables the centerpiece of the meal rather than a side dish. Cook a stir-fry or a "bed" of sautéed greens with fish or chicken on top.

Cook extra meals and freeze, or use leftovers for other meals and snacks. Some children are better eaters at breakfast or lunch, so try using vegetables during these meals. Send a favorite chili, stew, or casserole to work or school in a stainless-steel thermos (see *Equipment* in Appendix C) with a bag of shredded cheese or other favorite topping. How nice to have a warm, nourishing meal in the middle of the day, especially in winter!

Soups are one of the best ways to include vegetables as well as other nutrient-dense real foods. Nothing compares to a fresh, homemade soup, which can be used for any meal. Soup for breakfast is a great way to start the day. Soups may require initial effort, but are inexpensive, packed with nutrients, and last for several meals. Learn a few basic recipes, make them several times, then start experimenting. Keep carrots, onions, celery, and garlic on hand and on the grocery list. Slice strips of dark leafy greens and add them just before serving. Try preparing soups on weekends and enjoy them for the week.

Get into the habit of using vegetable toppings for sandwiches, wraps, and pockets. For the more determined, puree vegetables to sneak into soups, sauces, and mashed potatoes—or even juice them for drinks and smoothies. Don't forget "veggie" muffins, breads, and pancakes. Carrot, pumpkin, sweet potato, and zucchini are typical favorites. Develop "get-rid-of-the-vegetables" strategies for leftovers and extras. Make a stir-fry or casserole at the end of the week or soup on the weekend before the next round of shopping.

Some find it helpful to plan and chop vegetables ahead of time. Cut vegetables may lose some nutrients when exposed to air, but that is better than not eating them at all. Having pre-cut vegetables on hand for snacks, appetizers, dipping, salads, sandwiches, soups, and meals dramatically increases the likelihood of their being used and eaten. Find a system which works for you: chop at night for the next day, in the morning, or throughout the day.

Fruits contain the natural sugar fructose. They are sweeter and tend to be easier to include. It is also easy to fall into the habit of buying the same ones all the time. Focus on variety, experimenting, and learning about eating seasonally (see chart p.48). Start squeezing, smelling, and buying. Sometimes you win; sometimes you learn a lesson. An A-to-Z reference book on hand might be helpful, especially when children pick out produce you have never seen before (see Appendix D).

Keep a bowl with seasonal fruit on the counter and berries in the refrigerator. If the fruit ripens before you are ready to eat it, place it front and center in the refrigerator to slow the ripening, or use it in a smoothie. Buy inexpensive overripe bananas to peel, bag, and freeze for smoothies or bread when you have time. Occasionally add fun and exotic fruits you do not normally buy. Keep bags of organic, frozen fruit in the freezer for smoothies, breads, or to thaw and eat in emergencies. This will also allow for more variety in winter. Canned, again, is a last choice but better than nothing. Select canned fruits packed in natural juices without syrup, sugars, dyes, or other additives.

Dried fruit is full of nutrients and often forgotten. Keep one or two bags on hand and rotate monthly. Choose a favorite (we like raisins, apricots, and figs) and something new to expand horizons. Use them for snacks, trail mix, or in breads, cookies, and hot cereals. Try to buy organic, dried fruit at the health food store. Most conventional dried fruits, along with pesticides, have been treated with the preservative sulfur dioxide. Sulfur dioxide keeps the fruit moist and colorful but can cause allergic reactions and destroys B vitamins.

Be aware that it is easy to get carried away eating dried fruit. It would be difficult to eat 10 whole apricots but easy to eat 10 dried with the same amount of sugar. Fruit juices are also concentrated sugars. Eat whole fruits. Drink water. Drinking extra water is also important as dried fruits will rehydrate when eaten. Be careful of dried fruits with coatings. Many are natural like honey, others are not. Fruits are sweet already. They do not need sweet coatings. Dried fruits can also stick to your teeth. Raisins are one of the most cavity-causing foods because the sugars stick to the enamel. They are still more nutritious than candy. Just brush your teeth afterward.

Originally, I was not fond of the idea of playing with food. But if making vegetable faces, zucchini grass, and broccoli trees encourages kids to eat their vegetables, it is fine with me. Try to be aware of children's developmental phases. They will naturally be wary of new foods during particular times, and reject foods they previously accepted. It can be frustrating, but be flexible, persistent, and keep the big picture in mind.

Whenever possible, involve children in the process of growing, choosing, and preparing produce. Probably one of the best ways to connect children with fresh fruits and vegetables is to plant a garden. It could be as simple as a few pots of tomato plants or as elaborate as large beds. When children are invested in planning, planting, caring, and harvesting, they tend to be invested in eating. Even try canning or freezing extra produce to help cut down on costs and provide more food year round. If this seems unrealistic for you, learn about seasonal produce, find a place to go "picking," and leave the rest to the experts.

Local farmstands, farmers' markets, and Community Supported Agriculture (CSA) farms are other great options. CSA farms are becoming increasingly popular. Most are run by small organic, or biodynamic, farmers who sell "shares" in the farms. Members stop by weekly to pick up their part of the harvest. It's a wonderful way to obtain fresh, organic produce and to learn about new foods. Individual farms operate differently, but most have newsletters which provide helpful recipes and suggestions (see Appendix B or E). If you are fortunate to live near farms or farmers' markets, visit often and bring the kids to help them to discover where food comes from (hint: not the store).

Storing: Look for loose produce that looks fresh, firm, and crisp. There should be no bruises, mold, or sprouting. Use a produce wash or a drop of dish soap and water to clean both organic and conventional produce. Peeling helps remove chemicals but also nutrients. Keep most fruit out on the counter or in a basket, and berries, grapes, and cut fruit in the refrigerator. Refrigerating dried fruit in sealed plastic or glass containers helps them last longer. Place vegetables in the crisper (vegetable bin) in the refrigerator (except for onions, garlic, potatoes, and squashes, which should be kept in a cool, dark place).

Under-ripe fruit can be placed in a paper bag to ripen more quickly (add a banana to accelerate the ripening process.) Sometimes, letting fruit ripen slowly out on the counter will provide fruit later in the week. If fruit reaches its peak before you are ready, place it in the refrigerator to extend it a few more days. If you have time, peel and freeze extra fruit, or use it in a smoothie.

I'm always amazed when I see someone with a strange vegetable or exotic fruit in a shopping cart. I want to follow them around, see what else they buy, and ask, "What do you do with that?" At this point, however, I refrain from shopper-stalking and limit myself to asking people for recipes in the check-out line.

Shifting Summary

Start with:

- *fresh vegetables and salad daily with dinner; use leftovers in eggs or for lunch*
- *dried fruit for snacks; make smoothies; vegetable snacks with dips*
- *vegetable breads, muffins, and pancakes (use extra pumpkin puree in pancake batter); stock up on produce (canned, if necessary)*

Shift to:

- *various vegetable families; serve dark leafy greens once a week*
- *soup once or twice a month; stew, chili, or slow-cooker recipes with fresh produce*
- *learn basic vegetable stir-fry, casserole, and pasta recipes*
- *MYOM with fresh, quality produce (pizzas and Mexican dishes)*

Most nutritious:

- *Learn about canning and / or freezing seasonal produce*
- *start a garden or consider joining a community farm (CSA)*
- *research natural food cooperatives, buying clubs, and mail order organic products*

Shopper's Guide to Pesticides in Produce from Environmental Working Group (more information can be found at www.foodnews.org)	
High Pesticide Foods (Buy Organic)	Low Pesticide Foods
Apples	Asparagus
Bell peppers	Avocados
Celery	Bananas
Cherries	Broccoli
Grapes (imported)	Cauliflower
Nectarines	Corn (sweet)
Peaches	Kiwi
Pears	Mangos
Potatoes	Onions
Red raspberries	Papayas
Spinach	Pineapples
Strawberries	Peas (sweet)

Table 6: Pesticides in Produce

FRUITS

What to Limit or Eliminate:
Heavily sprayed fruits; waxed fruits
Fruits dried with sulfur dioxide
Canned fruits (except for emergencies), especially those in syrup

What to Add or Increase:
Organic, unwaxed, local fruits in season; local, in-season; frozen organic

Fruit	Description and Uses
Apple	Fiber, cholesterol-lowering pectin; >7,000 varieties; baking, applesauce
Apricot	Protein, iron, calcium, vitamin A, zinc, and beta carotene; also dried
Avocado	Fat, fiber, vitamin E; buy firm, when softened, slice, "de-pit," scoop out flesh
Banana	Potassium; great for smoothies and baby food
Blueberry	Vitamin C, manganese, and antioxidant; baking, jams, smoothies
Cantaloupe	Vitamin C, beta carotene, potassium; try honeydew and other melon varieties
Cherry	Iron and beta carotene; baking, jams; also try dried cherries
Fig	Iron, calcium, fiber, folic acid; also dried
Grapefruit	Low calorie, high fiber, vitamin C; also lemons, limes, clementines, tangerines
Grape	Antioxidant anthocyanin, vitamins A, B-complex, and C; raisins (dried)
Kiwi	Vitamin C, magnesium, and potassium
Mango	Vitamin A and C; peel and eat yellow flesh surrounding large, oval-shaped seed
Orange	Vitamin C, calcium, pectin fiber (white membrane has bioflavonoids)
Papaya	Vitamin A and C, enzyme papain aids digestion; try also guava
Peach	Vitamins A and C, calcium; baking, jams; also try nectarines
Pear	Pectin fiber, potassium, and boron; eases constipation
Pineapple	Manganese, vitamin C, and digestive enzymes
Plum	Vitamin C; also try dried plums (prunes)

Pomegranate	Potassium, phytonutrients; tart, juicy seeds sink in water (discard floating pith)
Raspberry	Fiber, folic acid, and zinc; antioxidants; also blackberries; fresh, baking, or jams
Strawberry	Vitamins A and C, and fiber; fresh, baking, or jams
Watermelon	Vitamins C and A, potassium
Tips:	
To ripen fruit quickly, store in paper bag with banana at room temperature	
How to Store:	
Citrus, melons, pineapple, and unripened fruit can be left on the counter or in cool, dry place	
Refrigerate grapes, berries, cut fruit, or ripened fruit	

Table 7 : Fruits

VEGETABLES	
What to Limit or Eliminate: Heavily sprayed vegetables; waxed vegetables Canned vegetables (except tomatoes and for emergencies)	
What to Add or Increase: Organic, unwaxed, local vegetables in season; local, in-season; frozen organic	
Vegetable	**Description and Uses**
Asparagus	Vitamins A, B-complex, C, and E, potassium, zinc, glutathione
Artichoke	Vitamins, potassium, iron, calcium, magnesium
Beet	Magnesium, iron, phosphorus; try smaller beet greens for salads
Broccoli	Vitamin C, calcium, selenium; cabbage family
Cabbage	Vitamins C, E, calcium, chlorophyll, minerals, antioxidants, and phytonutrients
Carrot	Vitamin A, carotenoids; try also parsnip
Celery	Vitamins A, B-complex, C, choline, and potassium
Cucumber	Silicon, water, digestive enzymes; cools, softens, clears skin
Eggplant	Potassium, water; large, purple, pear-shaped plant with sponge-like quality
Green Bean	Vitamins A and B-complex, calcium, and potassium
Kohlrabi	Vitamin C, potassium, fiber; peel, slice, steam or stir-fry
Lettuce	Butterhead, iceberg, loose-leaf, mesclun, radicchio, romaine; magnesium, silicon
Mushroom	Protein, vitamin B, and zinc; try other varieties
Onion	Lily family (leeks, garlic); antioxidants, antibacterial, anticancer agents
Peppers	Sweet peppers and other varieties; nightshade family
Potato	Tuber; nightshade family; manganese, chromium, selenium, molybdenum
Pumpkin	Vitamin A, potassium; helps to regulate blood sugar
Squash	Summer (crookneck, zucchini) and winter; vitamins A and C, potassium, calcium

Vegetable	Description and Uses
Sweet potato	Tuber; vitamins A and C, calcium, and carotenoids; also yams
Tomato	Nightshade family; vitamins A, B, and C, potassium, and phytochemicals
Tips: Onions cause potatoes to sprout (store separately) Cut greens off root vegetables (to drain moisture) before storing	
How to Store: Vegetable drawer in refrigerator (except onions, potatoes, roots, and tomatoes)	

Table 8 : Vegetables

FRUIT AND VEGETABLE FAMILIES	
Fruits	**Description and Uses**
Berries	Vitamins C, pectin, phytonutrients; blackberries, blueberries, rasberries, strawberries
Citrus	Vitamin C, potassium, (pith contain bioflavonoids); clementine, grapefruit, lemon, lime, oranges, tangerine, uglifruit
Melons	Beta-carotene, potassium; canary, cantaloupe, casaba, crenshaw, honeydew, watermelon
Vegetables	**Description and Uses**
Cruciferous	Calcium, magnesium, iron, vitamins A and C, anticarcinogenic (anti-cancerous) phytonutrients (especially dark leafy greens); arugula, beet greens, bok choy, broccoli, brussels sprouts, cabbage, cauliflower, chard, collards, daikon, endive, kale, kohlrabi, mizuna, mustard greens, watercress
Leafy Greens	Potassium, vitamins B and C, magnesium, phosphorus, iron, fiber; Arugula, beet greens, bok choy, chard, collards, endive, kale, mizuna, mustard greens, spinach, watercress
Roots and Tubers	Fiber, potassium, beta carotene, vitamin C; beets, burdock, carrots, celery root, daikon, fennel, onion, parsnip, potato, radish, rutabaga, sweet potato, turnip, yam
Squash (summer)	Vitamins A and C, potassium, and calcium; pattypan, scallop, yellow (crookneck), zucchini
Squash (winter)	Vitamins A and C, potassium, iron, riboflavin, and magnesium; acorn, butternut, chayote, pumpkin, spaghetti

Table 9 : Fruit and Vegetable Families
*choose from different families (especially those in season) for a variety of nutrients (some vegetables are classified in more than one category)

SEASONAL CHART*			
Spring	**Summer**	**Fall**	**Winter**
Artichokes	Apricots	Apples	Avocados
Asparagus	Arugula	Arugula	Bananas
Avocados	Bananas	Bananas	Broccoli
Bananas	Beans	Beets	Cabbage
Broccoli	Beets	Broccoli	Carrots
Cabbage	Blackberries	Brussels sprouts	Celery
Carrots	Blueberries	Cabbage	Collard
Collard	Cabbage	Carrots	greens
greens	Chard	Cauliflower	Grapefruits
Leafy greens	Cherries	Chard	Kale
Leeks	Corn	Cranberries	Kiwi
Mustard	Cucumbers	Cucumbers	Leeks
greens	Eggplant	Garlic	Mushrooms
Oranges	Figs	Grapes	Mustard
Papaya	Garlic	Kale	greens
Peas	Grapes	Leeks	Oranges
Pineapples	Green beans	Leafy greens	Pears
Rhubarb	Kohlrabi	Mushrooms	Rutabaga
Spinach	Leafy greens	Mustard greens	Spinach
Strawberries	Mangos	Oranges	Sweet potato
	Melons	Pears	Winter
	Nectarines	Peppers	squash
	Okra	Pomegranates	
	Peaches	Potatoes	
	Peppers	Pumpkins	
	Plums	Rutabagas	
	Radishes	Sweet potatoes	
	Raspberries	Winter squash	
	Summer squash		
	Tomatoes		

Table 10 : Seasonal Foods Chart
*varies according to region—become familiar with local, seasonal produce for variety and peak nutrients

Nuts, Seeds, and Oils

"Fats in nature are good, but what we have done to good natural fats—deep frying and processing them from their natural state into oils—damages human physiology."
Diana Schwarzbein, MD and Nancy Deville,
The Schwarzbein Principle

For many people, their only exposure to nuts and seeds are peanuts, which do not count because they are actually a legume. Most, however, do use oils which are primarily extracted from seeds. There has been much debate over fats and oils (fats in liquid state.) Are they healthy? Which ones? How much? "Low-fat" and "No fat" are popular advertising slogans and lead us to believe fat is unhealthful. But fats are essential and necessary for the body to function properly. Oils, though, are not whole foods. Their original source is in seeds (grains, nuts, and legumes), fruits (avocados and olives), and fish. Extracting, refining, and cooking with oils can damage them. (The issues surrounding oils are discussed in this section.)

Benefits: Nuts and seeds are among the most nutritious foods in the world. They are high in fat, protein, essential fatty acids, fiber, B vitamins, folic acid, calcium, potassium, magnesium, phosphorus, iron, zinc, vitamin E, and selenium. The oils in these seeds provide us with energy, help the body use vitamins, build healthy cells, improve brain function, contribute to healthy skin and hair, make hormones, cushion organs, and help us feel full and satisfied.

Issues: Nuts and seeds in their original, whole form are relatively nutritious and stable. Once shelled, chopped, or ground, however, the oils in these plants begin to oxidize and become rancid (spoil). Also, toxins tend to settle in fats, so organic is a more healthful choice. The use of oils extracted from plants raises several issues: problems with extraction, refining, hydrogenation, maintaining a healthy omega-3 to omega-6 ratio, and appropriate use of fats for cooking.

The oils extracted from nuts and seeds are primarily polyunsaturated. They are very delicate and easily damaged by heat, oxygen, and light. It is important to purchase oils which have been extracted properly, preferably unrefined. There are two ways to extract oil: expeller (or mechanical) pressure or solvent extraction. Expeller-pressed oils are squeezed from the seed, while solvent extracted oils use hexane or other petroleum solvents to remove the oil. The oil-solvent solution is then heated to evaporate the solvent, but residues may be left behind. Cold-pressed oils are expeller pressed in an environment of less than 120 degrees Fahrenheit. Look for "100 percent mechanically pressed" or "100 percent expeller-pressed" unrefined oils for the most nutrients and full, natural flavors.

After extraction, oils can be refined to remove strong flavors, odors, and impurities. Refining makes for a milder taste and smell, and it enables the oil to be used at a higher heat. Some refining processes use chemicals for degumming, alkali refining, bleaching, hydrogenating, and deodorizing. Most of the nutrients have been removed or destroyed and, in the case of hydrogenation, damaging compounds created.

Hydrogenation is the chemical process of changing natural oils into semi-solid or solid fats. These are unnatural and contain harmful trans-fatty acids. Trans-fats are not metabolized in our bodies like natural fats and can result in a deformed cellular structure. Read labels and eliminate any foods containing hydrogenated or partially hydrogenated oils.

Essential fatty acids perform key bodily functions and are vital to our health. They cannot be manufactured by the body so they must be obtained from the diet. There are two essential fatty acid families: omega-6 fatty acids or linoleic acid (LA) and omega-3 fatty acid or alpha-linolenic acid (ALA). Our ancestors obtained these from eating plants, seeds, fish, and other plant-eating animals. They maintained a healthy 1:1 ratio of these two essential fatty acids. Our modern diet, however, is excessively high in omega-6 fatty acids (prominent in many plant oils except walnut and flax) and dangerously lacking in omega-3 fatty acids (as are grain-fed animals), ranging anywhere from 20:1 to 40:1. This imbalance disrupts prostaglandins, hormone-like compounds that regulate vital body functions. Consuming too many plant oils magnifies this distortion. It is most desirable to shift back to a more healthful 1:1 ratio by decreasing the omega-6 fatty acids found in most processed plant oils and increasing omega-3 fatty acids contained in flax seeds,* fish oils, and grass-fed animal products.

As discussed earlier, there are three types of fats: saturated, mono-unsaturated, and polyunsaturated. The difference in their "saturation" determines the solidity of the fat at room temperature. The more satu-rated fats, like butter and coconut oil, are solid at room temperature. Although criticized for high calories and cholesterol, these are the most stable fats, able to resist damage from heat and oxidation, and best for high-temperature cooking and baking.

Oils made up of primarily monounsaturated fats, olive, canola, and sunflower, can withstand moderate heat and be used for low-tem-perature cooking. Olive oil, easily found expeller pressed and unrefined, is prominent in Mediterranean diets and praised for its many health benefits. It is sold in three grades: pure, virgin, and extra virgin. The most desirable and least damaged is extra virgin olive oil. It is an excel-lent choice for salad dressings, marinades, and low-temperature sautéing and cooking.

If oil begins to form ripples (waves), it is too hot. If it smokes, free radicals have been created and it is toxic. Throw it out and start over. Advanced glycoxidation end products (AGEs) occur when glucose and fats are cooked together at high heat. Recent research suggests AGEs are implicated in complications of diabetes, heart disease, and overall aging. Foods with fat or cooked in fat are more at risk of developing AGEs, especially when cooked at high heat. Cooking at lower temperatures and adding moisture lowers the development of AGEs. The best cooking methods are poaching, boiling, or sautéing. The most dangerous are broiling, grilling, and frying.

Polyunsaturated fats, found in walnut, safflower, and flax oils*, are also the most delicate. These plant oils contain essential fatty acids the body needs, but they should not be exposed to heat, light, or oxygen.

Unfortunately, most are already damaged during the extracting and re-fining processes, which are compounded when they are mistakenly used for cooking. This creates more trans-fatty acids and free radicals which damage the body on a cellular level. Try to find quality polyunsaturated oils; they are best used for dressings and marinades that will not be cooked, or as a flavoring on top of cooked vegetables and grains.

> **Flaxseed is one of the richest sources of omega-3 fatty acids. Supplementing with ground flax seeds or flax seed oil can help increase the essential fatty acid omega-3. Grind small amounts (a coffee grinder works well; use immediately) to add to yogurt, smoothies, or hot cereals. Flax oil, purchased in dark, refrigerated bottles, can also be added to foods or taken directly. Use within six to eight weeks. Quality fish and fish oils (see Fish section) and grass-fed animals (see Poultry and Eggs, Dairy, and Meat sections) are also rich sources of omega-3 fatty acids.*

Shifting: First, throw away old, rancid nuts and seeds, anything with a bitter smell or taste. Chopped nuts and seeds, especially, spoil quickly. Replace them with fresh bags, ideally whole and organic, and store them in the refrigerator for up to three months or freeze. Use them for snacks, trail mix, salads, breads, cookies, casseroles, and other baked products. They can be purchased shelled or unshelled, raw or roasted, coated or plain. Some recommend buying unshelled nuts because oxidation begins quickly, but shelling nuts can be quite time consuming (although a fun job for kids.) Do not buy or eat nuts that taste bitter or have dark spots. They are rancid and can cause liver and other oxidative damage.

Next, read labels and replace any products containing hydrogenated oil, partially hydrogenated oil, or vegetable shortening. This includes margarine, processed foods, baked goods, cookies, crackers, and most salad dressings and spreads. It can be a shock to see how many products, especially snacks foods, contain hydrogenated oils. (Ever wonder why those cookies and crackers seem to last forever in your cabinet?) It can also be a shock when products with natural oils spoil quickly. You don't want to eat rancid products either. Find out what you really eat and develop a routine for rotating healthful foods through your house.

Replace old bottles of vegetable oil with unrefined, extra-virgin olive oil for dressings and low-temperature cooking, sesame or peanut oil for medium temperatures, and (gasp!) butter, clarified butter (ghee), or quality, unrefined coconut oil for high-temperature cooking and baking. It is better to use a natural, saturated fat able to withstand high temperatures than a "healthful" unsaturated fat which becomes damaged and transforms into a trans fat. Butter contains fat-soluble vitamins and important minerals and is generally used in small amounts (see **Dairy** section.) If the rest of your diet is nutritious and does not contain processed, convenience foods, this amount of saturated fat is minimal and healthful.

Purchase small, dark bottles of flax oil in the refrigerated section of the supermarket or health food store. Drizzle it on salads, grains, pasta, and vegetables, or take it straight by the teaspoon. Get into the habit of putting the flax bottle out on the table with the salad dressings at dinner. Others put it in oatmeal, smoothies, or drizzle it on toast. It is very delicate, so never use it for cooking, always refrigerate, and use within a few weeks.

Nuts and seeds can also be ground into butters. Peanuts, used to make the ever-popular peanut butter, are actually legumes. Many conventional brands add hydrogenated oil to keep a uniform consistency, and sugar. Peanuts are also prone to developing the toxic mold aflatoxin and, as a result, the crops are heavily sprayed with pesticides. Valencia peanuts are grown in drier climates and less prone to mold. Look for brands made with Valencia peanuts without added sugar and hydrogenated oils, try organic, or switch to other flavorful nut butters.

Nut butters made from cashews, almonds, and other nuts and seeds are becoming increasingly popular. Almond butter is great for dips and spreads and high in calcium (eight times higher than peanut butter and four times more than milk). Cashew butter tends to be thicker but great for spreading on hearty bread and thickening smoothies and soups. Sesame seed butter (tahini) and hummus (from chickpeas and tahini) are other flavorful spreads. Health food stores and now many conventional grocery stores carry these healthful variations.

The oil in natural nut butters can separate, and mixing it back in can be messy. Some suggest storing the jar upside down before opening. I use the highly advanced, technical procedure of sticking a kitchen knife in the middle and twisting until the oil begins to blend. Then I stir gently and store in the refrigerator.

Nuts can be difficult to digest and a choking hazard. Most health experts recommend waiting until children are 18 months old to begin nut butters and three years to try whole nuts. Peanuts and tree nuts are also common allergens. Those with a family history may be more susceptible.

Soaking nuts and seeds overnight can make them easier to digest and the nutrients more available and easier to assimilate. They can also be sprouted. Sprouting seeds produces vitamin C and increases the vitamin B content as well as the enzymes which aid digestion. While these may seem to be unrealistic suggestions now, it may be an area to explore in the future. Just planting a seed.

Storing: Nuts and seeds should be purchased fresh and stored in sealed containers in the refrigerator for up to three months. Buy an old favorite and a new variety every month, rotating as you do with dried fruits. Keep oils in the refrigerator, close bottles tightly, and use within a few months, flax oil within six to eight weeks. Olive and sesame oils contain vitamin E, a natural preservative, and can be stored in a cool, dark place. (They also solidify in the refrigerator and need to be left out or run under warm water to be liquefied again. This can be time consuming and frustrating. Buy small bottles and use quickly or transfer to a wide-mouth jar and scoop out solidified oil as needed.) Nuts, seeds, and unrefined, organic oils can be found in the natural food section of some grocery stores, health food stores, mail-order, or through buying clubs.

The most natural and nutritious way to obtain healthful plant oils is while they are still in the plant. Eat whole nuts, seeds, grains, and other foods containing oils before they are extracted. Organic, unrefined flax, olive, and sesame oil, as well as butter, clarified butter, or coconut oil, should cover most of your health and cooking needs.

Shifting Summary

Start with:

- *replacing rancid nuts and seeds; use fresh for snacks, salads, and baked goods*
- *replacing refined "vegetable" and hydrogenated oils (margarine and shortening)*
- *finding a quality brand of peanut butter, free of sugars and hydrogenated oil*

Shift to:

- *new nut butters for sandwiches, snacks, dipping, or in smoothies*
- *quality olive and sesame oil for dressings and low-temperature cooking*
- *butter, clarified butter, or unrefined coconut oil for medium to high-heat cooking*

Most nutritious:

- *flax seed oil on salads, pasta, toast, or oatmeal; keep refrigerated*
- *organic nuts, seeds, and oils (find in health food stores, food co-ops, or by mail)*
- *grinding fresh nut butters; soaking and/or sprouting nuts and seeds*
- *low heat cooking methods (poaching or boiling)*

NUTS and SEEDS

What to Limit or Eliminate:
Rancid nuts and seeds (spoiled): bitter taste, odor, dark edges or spots,
    chopped and exposed to air over a long period of time
Conventional nut butters with hydrogenated oils, sugar, or other additives

What to Add or Increase:
Fresh, raw, whole nuts and seeds (organic, if possible)
Fresh, organic nut and seed butters: almond, cashew, macadamia,
    sunflower, and sesame

Nuts	Description and Uses
Almond	Potassium, magnesium, calcium, and other vitamins and minerals; try butter
Brazil Nut	Potassium, phosphorus, calcium, and sulfur
Cashew	Magnesium, phosphorus, potassium, and vitamin A; try butter
Chestnut	Higher carbohydrate and lower fat than most nuts
Coconut	Technically a fruit; high in saturated fat; try milk, meat (dried or flaked), and oil
Filbert	Hazelnut; potassium, phosphorus, sulfur, and calcium
Macadamia	Sweet flavor; 70 percent fat
Peanut	Technically a legume; common food allergen; protein, fat, B vitamins, and iron
Pecan	Hickory family; phosphorus, potassium, and vitamin A
Pine Nut	Pignolia; fat, vitamins, and minerals; use in salads and pesto
Pistachio	Green color; protein, calcium, vitamin A, iron, and potassium
Walnut	Omega-3 fatty acids, zinc, calcium, potassium, magnesium, and vitamin A
Seeds	**Description and Uses**
Alfalfa	Vitamins A, E, D, and K; popular for sprouting
Flax	Healthy oil and omega-3 fatty acids; aids digestion; laxative effect

Pumpkin	Iron, zinc, phosphorus, and vitamin A
Sesame	Calcium, potassium, phosphorus, magnesium, and vitamin A; used in tahini
Sunflower	Potassium, phosphorus, silicon, calcium, and vitamin A

Tips:
To help mix in oil which has separated in nut butters, stir and refrigerate
A bitter smell or taste means the nuts have become rancid and should not
    be eaten
Valencia peanuts are grown in dry climates and are less susceptible to toxic
    mold aflatoxin
Sprouting increases nutrients and digestibility

How to Store:
Small amounts, whole, shelled in tightly sealed container in refrigerator
    for three to four months
Freeze up to a year
Unshelled are more protected and can last up to a year in cool, dry place

Table 11 : Nuts and Seeds

PLANT OILS

What to Limit or Eliminate:

Hydrogenated oils: unnatural transformation of liquid oils to solid form (trans fats); found in margarine, vegetable shortening, convenience foods, crackers, and other snack foods

Trans-fatty acids: due to high heat during refining or improper cooking (see "Tips")

Refined oils: "solvent extracted" with chemical residues, degummed, bleached, deodorized

Oxidized oils: rancid after exposure to light and oxygen

What to Add or Increase:

Plants in their natural state with oils intact: nuts, grains, seeds, beans, olives, and avocados

Expeller-pressed, unrefined plant oils

Plant Oil	Description and Uses
Canola	From *Can*adian rapeseed; high pesticide-use crop, buy organic; usually refined for baking and medium-heat cooking
Coconut	Tropical oil; high in saturated fat; most stable oil; buy unrefined; contains lauric acid and no trans-fats; use in baking and high-heat cooking
Corn	Look for unrefined; low to medium-heat cooking
Flax	High in EFAs and omega-3 fatty acids (also hemp seed); least stable oil; refrigerate or freeze; use on salads, grains, vegetables, in smoothies, or as a supplement
Grapeseed	Medium-high heat cooking; look for chemical-free processing (also expeller-pressed avocado oil)
Olive	Flavorful, stable oil; natural antioxidants, long shelf life; extra virgin (first pressing) most healthful; "pure" is refined; use in salad dressings, marinades, low-heat cooking
Palm	Also palm kernel oil; tropical oil; saturated fat, most stable oil; buy unrefined; use high-heat cooking; avoid refined oil and its products
Peanut	Stable oil; high pesticide-use crop, buy organic (hard to find); sesame and olive better choices; medium-heat cooking

Safflower	Look for unrefined; low-heat cooking and dressings; also high-oleic, more stable oil
Sesame	Favorful, stable oil; natural antioxidants provide longer shelf life; moderate heat cooking; also toasted for more intense flavor
Sunflower	Look for expeller pressed, chemical-free refining; unstable oil; refrigerate; use on salads, grains, vegetables; also high-oleic, more stable oil
Walnut	Look for expeller pressed, chemical-free refining; small amount of omega-3 fatty acids; unstable oil; refrigerate; use on salads, grains, vegetables

Tips:

Use more stable (saturated) fats for high-temperature cooking; olive or sesame oil for lower temperature cooking (see cooking chart p. 60); "ripples" indicate it is becoming too hot

Puncture a vitamin E capsule and squeeze contents into oil to help preserve and add antioxidants

Flax oil remains liquid in the freezer; placing in the freezer will extend shelf life

How to Store:

Small quantities in opaque glass containers in refrigerator (except coconut oil)

In tightly closed containers, use in one to two months (except olive and sesame oil—up to a year)

Use flax oil in six to eight weeks or freeze; hemp seed oil six to twelve weeks or freeze

Table 12 : Plant Oils

COOKING WITH FATS and OILS*		
Heat	**Fats& Oils**	**Description and Uses**
No Heat	Flax Fish Oils Therapeutic Oils •Black currant •Borage •Evening primrose	High in essential fatty acids (EFAs), particularly omega-3s; buy fresh, mechanically pressed, unrefined, organic, if possible, and refrigerate; use as supplements or cold in dressings and dips
Low Heat	Unrefined Oils •Virgin olive •Safflower •Sesame •Sunflower	Full seed flavors and nutrients; high in essential fatty acids, particularly omega-6 (except olive oil); use with high omega-3 oils to help maintain proper EFA balance; use in dressings, dips, sauces, or light sautéing
Medium Heat	Refined or semi-refined oils •Avocado •Canola •Sesame •Peanut	Higher in monounsaturated fatty acids; more refined oils can withstand higher heat; use for baking, sautéing, or light stir-frying
High Heat	Clarified Butter (ghee) Butter Tropical Oils •Coconut •Palm High Oleic oils •Safflower •Sunflower	Higher in saturated fatty acids, low in EFAS, more stable for cooking; clarified butter has the milk protein (whey) removed and a higher smoke point; use small amounts of unhydrogenated fats and oils for baking, sautéing, stir-frying, searing, or browning

Table 13 : Cooking with Fats and Oils

* Do not heat oil to its smoking point. If oil smokes, it is damaged and free radicals have been created. Discard the oil and begin again.

Legumes

"Looked at in total, the seed is the spark of life, a living and perfect food with all the elements necessary for life." —Paul Pitchford, *Healing with Whole Foods*

I confess I was an adult before I realized legume is another word for bean. Legumes grow on vines and are contained in pods which split open when mature. Once referred to as "poor man's meat," these seeds (nuts, grains, and legumes are all seeds) contain the potential to grow into plants and are a concentrated storehouse of nutrients and one often neglected.

Benefits: Legumes (beans, peas, and lentils) are very nutrient dense, containing protein, complex carbohydrates, soluble and insoluble fiber, as well as potassium, calcium, iron, zinc, folic acid, B vitamins, and phytonutrients. Darker-skinned beans such as black, pinto, and kidney actually have higher levels of antioxidants than lighter-skinned beans but all are nutritious and beneficial. They are low in fat, calories, and price, and are easy to find. Beans can be purchased either dried or canned. Dried beans retain more of their nutrients but need to be cooked.

Issues: Legumes are natural, unrefined, whole foods with few issues surrounding them. The complex sugars in beans can be difficult to digest, causing gas and intestinal discomfort. If you choose dried beans, it is important to prepare them properly. Soybeans, a nutrient-dense legume popular in many Asian cultures for thousands of years, are often subject to intensive refining in our modern society.

Beans contain difficult-to-digest complex sugars. When these sugars are broken down by bacterial enzymes in the intestines, they can cause gas and intestinal discomfort. Soaking beans prior to cooking helps predigest sugars and also neutralizes phytic acid, making nutrients more digestible and easily absorbed. Eating smaller quantities of beans and gradually increasing the amount until the body adjusts can also help manage digestibility.

There are various ways to soak beans. Place dried beans in water three to four times their volume for eight hours or overnight (during hot weather, place in refrigerator). Discard the soaking liquid, add fresh water two inches above beans, boil for 10 minutes, then cover and simmer until tender. Others recommend boiling beans for three minutes then removing them from the heat for three to four hours. Discard the water, rinse the beans, add new water, and proceed with cooking. Canned beans do not need to be soaked but are often canned with salt, sugar, and other additives. Read labels and consider rinsing before use.

Soybeans are high in protein, unsaturated fats, fiber, B vitamins, folic acid, potassium, calcium, zinc, and iron as well as the plant estrogen isoflavone. They also contain phytic acid, which can interfere with mineral absorption and trypsin inhibitors, which make proteins difficult to digest. Traditional cultures have learned to manage these issues by cooking and fermenting soybeans to produce foods such as miso (a fermented soybean paste), soy sauce, and tempeh.

Our society, however, uses soy as an inexpensive ingredient in many prepared, packaged, and restaurant foods. Soybeans are one of the most popular crops (second only to wheat.) They are cheap, easy to grow, a high pesticide-use crop, and often genetically engineered.* These soybeans are not fermented to manage trypsin inhibitors and phytates, but processed into refined flour, oil, soy protein isolates, and other products to be used as fillers, binders, and meat extenders. There are also concerns about the effects of soy estrogens (isoflavones), especially in infant formula. (For more information about concerns with soy infant formulas see Appendix B).

We have recently observed a glut of positive then negative soy publicity. It has gone from being a "cure-all" to having a "darker side." Now we can put soy in its rightfully balanced place along with other nutritious products. As with other real foods, look for organic, unrefined quality soy products, managed and prepared properly, without undesirable additives. Dr. Thyr's soy rule: If you have none, have some. If it is your main source of protein, cut down.

> **My husband and I used to be avid fans of the weed killer Round Up. We declared war on any weed and always won. Soon after, I read an article stating the Monsanto Company, the makers of Round Up, had developed genetically engineered Roundup Ready soybeans. These soybeans allowed farmers to spray Round Up weed killer on their crops, killing the undesirable plants but not the resistant soybeans. While this may seem like a great advancement for soybean production, my first thought was, "I am consuming Round Up." I have been buying organic soy products ever since. Genetically engineered (GE) and genetically modified organisms (GMOs) do not have to be labeled. Buying organic or contacting the manufacturuer are, currently, the only ways to ensure you are not consuming Roundup Ready soybeans or other GE or GMO foods.*

Shifting: If you have few or no beans in your diet, buy canned and use them sprinkled on a salad, have baked beans as a side dish, or put some in a soup. Make a bean dip, have chili, or prepare your favorite Mexican meal which includes beans.

Happy mediums between canned and dried beans are lentils and split peas. These are very nutritious, easily digested, and do not need soaking. Use them in a soup by bringing it to a boil, then simmer and cover for 45 minutes to an hour. When puréed, they add a thick, creamy texture to soups as well as protein and fiber.

Begin to experiment with quality soy products. Tofu (soybean curd) is available in different densities (extra firm, firm, or soft/silken) depending on your cooking needs. Try tofu in a dip (soft,) smoothie (firm), or in a stir-fry (extra firm.) Tofu absorbs the flavors of surrounding foods. Prepare it with other flavorful ingredients or marinate it prior to use.

Finally, develop a system to use dried beans which works for you. Use the soak-overnight method or the boil-remove-from-heat method and let sit for several hours. Always change the soaking water to help eliminate the complex sugars which cause gas. Cooking times vary greatly depending on type, age, and quality. Add water as needed and test for doneness toward the end of cooking time. Using a slow cooker or pressure cooker are other options. Pressure cooking reduces the time and water needed to prepare beans while preserving nutrients, flavor, and texture. Keep experimenting with soy products and make them a balanced part of a varied diet as you do other legumes.

Storing: Store uncooked, dried beans in a tightly sealed container in a cool, dry place for a year. They may toughen with age and require longer cooking times. (They also look nice and pretty all lined up in mason jars on the counter or in the pantry.) Cooked beans will last up to five days in the refrigerator and up to six months in the freezer. So cook extra to have on hand.

Store tofu, tempeh, and miso in the refrigerator and refer to "sell by" date. Tofu is usually sold in water-filled vacuum packs or aseptic brick packages. Once opened, leftover tofu should be submerged in water, covered, and stored in the refrigerator. Change the water daily and tofu will last for up to one week. It can also be frozen for up to five months.

Shifting Summary

Start with:
- *canned beans: rinsed, sprinkled on salads (chick peas or kidney beans)*
- *using baked or refried beans as a side dish*
- *making chili, burritos, or other beans meals; using canned beans in soup*

Shift to:
- *lentil and split pea soups (no soaking required)*
- *bean spreads and dips: hummus or white bean*
- *tofu in a smoothie or stir-fry*

Most nutritious:
- *soaking dried beans and cooking; try a three-bean salad, rice and beans, or casserole*
- *experimenting with other soy products: miso, tempeh, tamari, and natto*
- *finding resources for quality, organic legumes*

LEGUMES	
What to Limit or Eliminate: Beans that are cracked, shriveled, or fuzzy (mold)	
What to Add or Increase: Dried beans Canned beans without additives	
Legume	**Description and Uses**
Adzuki (aduki)	Small, dark, red; calcium, iron, phosphorus, potassium, and vitamin A
Black Beans (turtle)	Robust flavor; popular in soups or "refried"
Black-eyed Pea	Distinctive black "spot;" quick cooking
Garbanzo (chickpea)	Potassium, calcium, iron, and vitamin A; used for hummus
Kidney	Red or white (cannellini); baked beans
Lentils	More than 50 varieties (brown, green, red); protein, calcium, sulfur, magnesium, potassium, and phosphorus; no soaking required
Lima	Potassium, phosphorus, vitamin A
Mung	Small green; popular in Asia; easy to digest
Peas	Calcium, potassium, phosphorus; chili, soups, stews, or with grains
Pinto	Vitamins A and B, calcium, potassium; snow and sugar snap
Split Peas	Green or yellow; no soaking required
White	Navy (smaller) and great northern
Soybean	Complete protein, iron, B vitamins, and isoflavones, edamame (green, immature soybeans); used to make tofu, tempeh, miso, and tamari (soy sauce); hard to digest; use fermented

Tips:
Rinse, remove debris, and any legumes with pin holes (bugs)
Replace soaking water to help reduce flatulence (pour off and refill one to three times)
Choose darker-skinned beans, which contain more antioxidants
Use pressure cooker to reduce cooking time
Remove any legumes that rise to top when soaking (harvested prematurely and shrunk)
Skim off foam while cooking
Choose similar size legumes to help them cook uniformly
How to Store:
Uncooked, dried beans in a tightly sealed container in a cool, dry place for a year or more
Tofu, tempeh, and miso in the refrigerator; use "sell by" date

Table 14 : Legumes

COOKING LEGUMES (Stovetop)

Directions: Rinse beans and place in large pot with required amount of liquid (3 cups for presoaked beans and 4 cups for unsoaked beans.) Bring to a boil, reduce heat and simmer, covered, until tender.

Bean (1 cup dry)	Cooking Time (presoaked)*	Cooking Time (unsoaked)	Yield
Adzuki	60 min.	120 min.	2 cups
Black Bean	90 min.	120 min.	2 cups
Black-eyed Pea	30-45 min.	45-60 min.	2 cups
Garbanzo (chick pea)	90-120 min.	120-180 min.	2 cups
Great Northern (navy)	60-90 min.	90-120 min.	2 cups
Kidney	60 min.	120 min.	2 cups
Lentil	no soaking req.	30-45 min.	1 ¼ cups
Lima	60 min.	90-120 min.	2 cups
Mung	60 min.	90 min.	2 cups
Pinto Bean	60-90 min.	90-120 min.	2 ¼ cups
Split Pea	no soaking req.	45-60 min.	2 cups
White Kidney (cannellini)	60-90 min.	120-180 min.	2 cups
Soybean	2-3 hours	3-4 hours	2 cups

*Presoaking (except lentils and split peas): rinse beans then cover with three to four times amount of water for eight hours or overnight. Drain off soaking water, add required amount of fresh liquid and cook for allotted time. Or use "quick cook" method: boil for thee minutes and let sit off heat for two to three hours.

** Using a pressure cooker greatly reduces the cooking time of beans while increasing nutrients and flavor. Beans can also be cooked in a slow cooker (crock pot) for eight to 12 hours, depending on the type of bean.

***Salt and acid (tomatoes and vinegar) toughen the skins of beans. Add at the end of cooking time.

****Add a piece of Kombu (a type of sea vegetable) while cooking to increase digestibility.

Table 15 : Cooking Legumes

Sweeteners

"The key to satisfying your sweet tooth without experiencing sugar's
troublesome health risks is to satisfy it naturally and intelligently...
doing so will help you enjoy the sweet things in life
without the bitter consequences."
Ann Louise Gittleman, Ph.D., *Get The Sugar Out*

Sweeteners are some form of sugar: glucose, fructose, sucrose malt-ose, lactose—anything ending in "-ose." They come from sugar cane, sugar beets, fruits, grains such as corn, barley, and rice, maple trees, and bees. Sweets are products made with sweeteners. We are born with a sweet tooth and it has recently gotten us into trouble. The average person in the U.S. consumes about 150 pounds of sugar a year (and less than eight pounds of beans.) As a result, we are experiencing the consequences in disrupted body chemistry and ill health. There are, however, more natural, nutritious forms of sweeteners and those that are highly refined or even artificial. As with other real foods, it is most desirable to use unrefined, natural sweeteners with nutrients. We do not need to abandon sweets but return to wholesome, nutritious sweeteners combined with other nutrient-dense foods to eat in moderation.

Benefits: Sugars are carbohydrates which supply the body with quick energy. Natural sweeteners may have trace amounts of vitamins, minerals, and enzymes, but the amounts are usually insignificant. Blackstrap molasses, however, contains calcium, iron, and chromium; raw honey contains enzymes; dark honey has high levels of antioxidants; and pure maple syrup has trace minerals brought up from deep roots of the tree. It is best to choose natural sweeteners which concentrate nutrients through boiling, reducing, and evaporation, such as molasses, grain syrups, maple syrup, and jams, rather than removing them.

Issues: The key issues with sweeteners are refining and overcon-sumption. Sugar cane is a mineral-hungry plant which often depletes fertile soil reserves. Fertilizers and pesticides are commonly used on this crop. The refining process involves shredding and pressing the plant to remove the juice. The juice is strained, neutralized, boiled, clarified, evaporated, and spun, separating the sucrose from the rest of the plant. With each step, the natural sweetener is further removed from its natural state and its nutrients. Nothing remains but sugar, calories, and negative health effects. These denatured sweeteners are then combined with other refined ingredients (white flour, hydrogenated oils, undesirable additives, and preservatives) and consumed in excessive amounts by society as baked goods, snacks, and other processed foods.

Health problems relating to excess sugar include fluctuating blood sugar levels (see Glycemic Index p.29), obesity, diabetes, ADHD, heart disease, and cancer. Excess sugar causes cavities, has been linked to mood swings, behavioral problems, addictive tendencies, slow immune function, and a host of other health problems from acne to ulcers. Sugars are high in calories, often referred to as "empty calories" because of lacking nutrients, but "negative calories" would be more appropriate. Sugars extract nutrients from our own reserves to be digested. They create an acid condition which consumes our body's minerals and results in calcium loss. These conditions can lead to further complications and disease.

So we now have a nutrient-less food, high in calories, with a host of health-related issues, and our society is consuming more of it than ever. It is natural to want to satisfy our sweet tooth, but we need to do it in more healthful ways. Switch to more wholesome, natural sweeteners and combine them with other nutritious ingredients to make pies, cookies, breads, fruit crisps, puddings, and ice cream. Eat them in moderation, enjoy them, and experience better health.

Shifting: Start with finding quality natural sweeteners. Fill the house with fresh fruit, dried fruit, jellies, and jams. These tend to be lower in sugar and higher in nutrients while satisfying that sweet tooth. Use spices and flavorings like cinnamon, nutmeg, and vanilla which add a sweet taste. Find a quality brand of dark honey and pure maple syrup. Try shifting to less-sweet sources on pancakes like jam, nut butter, or applesauce. The fat in butter and the fiber in fruit pulp also slows digestion and releases sugar into the blood stream more steadily.

Next, try removing highly refined and artificial sweeteners such as high fructose corn syrup, aspartame, and saccharin. Artificial sweeteners are not recognized by the body and should be avoided. Watch for hidden sugars. Cold cereals are notorious for added sugar, but it is also in peanut butter, meats, yogurt, ketchup, and bread crumbs. Read labels and look for the "-ose." Sodas, especially, should be removed. They offer no nutrient value and contain phosphoric acid, which can interfere with absorption of nutrients, particularly calcium.

Finally, keep switching, reducing, and moving to less-sweet products. Experiment with natural sweeteners. They may require adjustments in cooking and tastes. I have tried maple sugar and grain syrups, but seem to find myself back using good, old, natural sugar. There is little nutritional difference between using natural sugar or white table sugar—a few trace nutrients and less bleaching, but it makes me feel better. I cut back the amount and make products with natural, nutrient-dense treats such as vegetable breads (carrot, zucchini, or pumpkin) and fruit desserts (apple crisp or oatmeal raisin cookies.) It is also acceptable for guests who want "sugar" for coffee or tea.

Health authorities often recommend eliminating sweeteners. They state sugars offer little or no nutrients, interfere with bodily functions, and are not necessary for the body to function in the first place. Like people from most societies, I enjoy sweet foods. They add to the pleasure and enjoyment of eating. I also enjoy spicy foods, sour foods, and the whole range of flavors and textures provided by real foods. Once again, it is a matter of balance, variety, and moderation.

Following my own advice isn't always easy. I focus on switching to more healthful sweets and reducing the overall amount in my diet, but when life gets busy or stressful, I usually head to the nearest form of chocolate. Chocolate is actually derived from the bean of the cacao tree. These beans are ground to make cocoa liquor, rich with cocoa butter. Solid cocoa liquor is sold as unsweetened chocolate and as cocoa powder when the cocoa butter is removed. These cocoa components are combined with sugar and other ingredients to make various chocolate products.

Chocolate contains antioxidant compounds, particularly dark chocolate, rich with flavonoids, phenols, and magnesium. It also contains the stimulants caffeine and theobromine, and oxalic acid, which can inhibit mineral absorption. Read labels and look for high-quality dark varieties with chocolate liquor and cocoa. Avoid those with hydrogenated oils replacing the cocoa butter and those with excess sugar. Some recommend carob as a chocolate alternative, but it is just not quite the same for me.

We try to reserve "sweet treats" for special occasions like birthday parties and holidays, have "desserts" occasionally after dinner, and keep lollipops for real emergencies. Although, there is usually a stash of decadent dark chocolate somewhere in the house for my emergencies. (I like to tell myself it's a good source of antioxidants.) Unfortunately, even small amounts of sugar can create cravings.

I find the more I learn about the negative effects of sugars, the more it motivates me to make changes. As I make changes to manage and balance my sugar intake, the better I feel. I don't deprive myself either. I just try to satisfy my sweet tooth in healthful, nutritious ways. (For more information see Appendix B.)

Storing: Most sweeteners can be stored in their original containers in a cool, dry place. Open containers of maple syrup should be stored in the refrigerator. If crystals form on honey and other syrups, place containers in warm water until they've dissolved.

Shifting Summary

Start with:
- *quality brands of jam, honey, and pure maple syrup*
- *natural sugar and reduced amounts in baking*
- *removing highly refined and artificial sweeteners (especially sodas)*

Shift to:
- *natural, sweet spices and flavorings such as cinnamon, nutmeg, and vanilla*
- *reading labels for hidden sugars; buying better-quality products*
- *baking with reduced amounts of sugar; including other nutrient-dense ingredients*

Most nutritious:

- *experimenting with other natural sweeteners; switch, reduce, remove*
- *reading informational material about the negative effects of sugar*
  (*see* Appendix B)
- *visit the health food store for greater variety of natural and organic sweeteners*

SWEETENERS	
What to Limit or Eliminate:	
Highly refined sweeteners: table sugar, brown sugar, fructose, corn syrup, artificial sweeteners: Aspartame, Saccharin, and others	
What to Add:	
Naturally sweet foods such as fruits Less-refined sweeteners: honey, maple syrup, grain syrups, and natural sugars	
Sweetener	**Description and Uses**
Date sugar	Ground, dehydrated dates; coarse; use in hot cereals, toppings, baking

Grain Syrups
  Barley Malt
 	
  Brown Rice
 	
  Sorghum
	
	Malted grain syrups and sugar: maltose; strong flavor (like molasses)
	Use in gingerbread and hearty flavored recipes; baking lighter, more delicate than barley malt; use like molasses
	From millet family; syrup like molasses; difficult to find

Fruit Products
  Conserves
  Concentrate
	
	Jam, jelly; may contain additives; spreads
	Usually refined juice; find quality, organic; baking

Honey*	Enzymes, darker, more minerals, flavor; unfiltered raw; flavors from flowers; spreads, baking, flavor drinks
Maple Syrup	Also maple sugar; minerals; graded flavor, color; grade B is least refined; choose formaldehyde-free buckets; use in cooking, baking, and spreads
Molasses	Liquid from refined sugar; minerals, thick syrup, strong flavor; Blackstrap: more nutrients; use in gingerbread, spice cookies, and hot cereals

Unrefined Sugar	Evaporated sugar cane juice; use as sugar

Tips:
Stevia: natural herb sweetener
Sugar alcohols (mannitol, sorbitol, xylitol); sugar substitutes made from adding hydrogen atoms to sugar; may be helpful for managing blood sugar levels; may cause intestinal distress
If crystals form, soak containers in warm water

How to Store:
Room temperature in a sealed glass jar/bag for one year
Refrigerate maple syrup after opening

Table 16 : Sweeteners

*never give honey to an infant younger than 12 months; bacteria, harmless to those one year and older, may cause botulism in babies

Animal Foods

*"As tens of thousands of people treat themselves to this wholesome,
nutritious, and delicious food [grass-fed animal products], they are
helping to save the farmers, the animals, the environment, and
their own health one meal at a time."*
—Jo Robinson, *Pasture Perfect*

Animals allowed to consume their natural diets in their natural environments produce the most nutrient-dense products. Like us, their bodies are designed to eat traditional diets and express natural behaviors. This reduces stress and disease, and helps them to develop into healthy animals. The products they produce are wholesome, natural, and nutritious.

Today, however, animals are often fattened and processed as quickly and inexpensively as possible at the expense of nutrition and nature. Concentrated Animal Feeding Operations (CAFOs), also referred to as factory farms, feed animals unnatural diets of grains and questionable materials such as animal byproducts and trash. Livestock are confined to small areas in which diseases spread and the need for antibiotics and other drugs is increased. Many animals are put on synthetic growth hormones and fed special diets to speed growth and time to market. The meat is processed quickly, often under unsafe, unsanitary conditions. This diet, stress, and environment can make animals sick and the products they produce unsafe and unhealthful.

Nutrient-dense animal foods are produced from animals allowed to eat their natural diet, live in their natural environment, express natural behaviors, and grow at their natural rate. Sustainable methods have a positive impact on the environment, ensure that animals are treated humanely, and produce healthful, nutritious, wholesome foods. Get real.

REFINED →→→→→→→→→→→→→→→→→→→→→→→→→→→→→→REAL		
Unnatural, unhealthful diets	More natural diets	Whole
Confined, crowded, and	More nutrient-	Nutrient-dense
stressed environment	dense foods and	Original form
Genetically altered or	products	Natural state
engineered	Natural	Clean
High-speed processing in	environment	Safe
unsanitary conditions	Less stress, disease	Nutritious
Hormone use	Fewer toxins in feed	
Antibiotic and other drug use	and environment	
Additives	Closer to original	
Preservatives	diet and	
	environment	

	REFINED →→→→→→→→→→→→→→→→→→→→→→→→→→→REAL		
FISH	Harvested in contaminated waters*	Farmed-raised in clean, spacious waters with quality feed	Fresh, clean, wild fish or quality farm-raised fish
	Farmed in crowded environments with poor-quality feed	Harvested in clean waters	Also flash frozen
	Canned with additives	Canned in water	
	Smoked with nitrites	Smoked without nitrites	
POULTRY	Battery (caged); or confined	Cage-free	Free-range poultry and eggs
	Selectively bred	Controlled, indoor environment with room to express natural behaviors	Grass-fed, grain-fed, allowed to forage (poultry is designed to survive on pasture as well as other forms of high-quality protein)
	Grain-fed and other questionable feed	Organic, grain-fed	
	Antibiotics and other drug use	Allowed some foraging	
	Products with additives		

	REFINED →→→→→→→→→→→→→→→→→→→→REAL		

DAIRY	Confined to feedlots
	Selectively bred
	High-protein
	    grains and other
	    questionable feed
	Antibiotics, hormones,
	    and other drugs
	Pasteurized/
	    homogenized
	Products with
	    additives
		Pasture-raised
		Grass-fed,
		    supplemented
		    with grains
		    when pasture
		    unavailable
		Pasteurized
		Organic products
			Raw dairy
			    products**
			Pasture-raised and
			    fed
			(**Raw milk is the
			    least processed
			    dairy product
			    but it is not
			    pasteurized
			    and may
			    carry disease-
			    producing
			    bacteria.)

RED MEAT	Factory-farmed
	Confined to feedlots
	Selectively bred
	High-protein
	    grains and other
	    questionable feed
	Antibiotics, hormones,
	    and other drugs
	Cured with nitrites
	Products with
	    additives
		Pasture-raised
		Grass-fed, grain
		    finished
		Organic products
		Naturally cured
		    products
			Grass-fed meats
			    and wild game
			Pasture-raised and
			    fed
			Grass-fed,
			    supplemented
			    when pasture is
			    unavailable

Table 17: Animal Foods

*The natural environment and diet of many fish has become contaminated. These are not "refined" but should be limited or avoided because of high toxin levels.

Fish

*"Widespread contamination of fish with toxic mercury, however,
has cast a shadow over the nutritional benefits of fish."* Ken Cook,
President of the Environmental Working Group

Fish are one of the most nutritious foods. People who consume
fish on a regular basis tend to live longer and experience less chronic
disease. It is also one of the most popular foods. Fish consumption rose
240 percent since 1960. As a result, the numbers of fish in our waters
are declining and the fish farming industry is growing to meet demand.
Consuming fish, however, poses several dilemmas.

Many wild species such as Chilean seabass, orange roughy, and
Atlantic halibut are over-fished and may not be able to recover. Other
fish are so contaminated with pollutants that health risks may outweigh
health benefits. And farmed fish can cause environmental problems and
may not be as nutritionally beneficial. Fortunately, quality fish choices
are still available.

Benefits: Fish include freshwater, saltwater, and shellfish (mollusks and crustaceans). There are wild and farmed varieties. Fish are an
excellent source of high-quality protein and a concentrated source of
minerals such as zinc, iron, magnesium, and phosphorus. They are low
in saturated fat and contain desirable omega-3 fatty acids, especially
fish from cold waters. They are easy to digest, providing more nutrition
with less work.

Issues: The main concerns with fish are over-fishing, contamination, and issues surrounding aquaculture (fish-farming). While over-
fishing is not a health problem, having adequate supplies of fish for the
future is a concern. Choosing fish with stable populations helps other
resources recover (see table p.82 and Appendix B).

Both wild and farmed fish can become contaminated from polluted
waters and improper handling procedures. Heavy metals such as mercury,

persistent organic pollutants (POPs) such as polychlorinated biphenyls (PCBs), and other chemical toxins have contaminated our air, soil, and water. Mercury from coal-burning power plant emissions, PCBs from synthetic fluids once used in electrical equipment, pesticides from agriculture (DDT and dioxin), and other toxic waste is in rain, runoff, or dumped into oceans, lakes, rivers, and coastal areas. Fish accumulate toxins from filtering polluted water or eating contaminated plants and other fish, increasing the concentration of toxins up the food chain to humans.

Mercury can cause a wide range of health problems from impaired vision and coordination to permanent neurological damage in fetuses and infants. The highest concentrations are found in longer-lived fish such as swordfish and tuna. PCBs were banned in 1977 because of possible links to cancer and other health issues. Even farmed carnivorous fish such as salmon, fed smaller, ground-up fish as feed, were found to have higher levels of PCBs than their wild counterparts.

The Food and Drug Administration (FDA) and the Environmental Protection Agency (EPA) advise sensitive populations (women who might become pregnant, women who are pregnant, nursing mothers, and young children) to avoid high-mercury fish (shark, swordfish, king mackerel, and tilefish), to eat up to two meals a week of fish and shellfish lower in mercury, and to check area advisories about the safety of fish caught in local waters. There are currently no restrictions on consuming farmed salmon.

Other health authorities are more stringent. Organizations such as the Environmental Working Group (EWG) and The Green Guide Institute include more fish on their list for sensitive populations to avoid and recommend limiting moderate-mercury and high-POP fish to one meal a month. While health authorities continue to debate limits, testing, and recommendations, we must decide what to put on our tables every day. Fish can be a nutritious food, but if you or your family is part of the "sensitive population" (even if you are not) it is important to understand the information and implications of eating contaminated fish (see table p.82 and Appendix B for more information).

Mollusks (clams, mussels, oysters, and scallops) and crustaceans (crabs, crawfish, lobsters, and shrimp) are typically shoreline and bottom-feeders and can be contaminated with bacteria from sewage and pollution around industrial and urban areas. Consuming raw mollusks is especially risky because of the possibility of viral or bacterial infection. It is important to obtain these from clean waters or to find quality farmed varieties.

Contamination can also occur from unsanitary conditions on boats or in processing plants, and from natural bacteria and parasites in fish that are not stored or cooked properly. Buy fish from a reputable vendor who knows where the fish came from and how it was handled. Continue to handle and store fish properly, and cook it thoroughly.

Fish-farming has become popular by providing a steady supply of fish at a lower cost. Nearly one-third of all fish consumed is farmed. Fish are raised in ponds, cages, pens, or manmade tanks and fed a controlled diet. In some instances, farmed varieties can be healthier than wild. Vegetarian fish (carp, catfish, and tilapia) and filter-feeders (clams, mussels, oysters, and scallops) benefit from clean water and food. On the other hand, farmed carnivorous fish such as shrimp and salmon can pose nutritional and environmental problems.

Crowded conditions can lead to stress and disease, resulting in the need for antibiotics or other chemical interventions. The diet of fish can vary greatly depending on the quality of feed and can change the nutritional makeup of the fish. Fish waste can cause pollution and escaped farm-fish can spread disease. Some in the fish-farming industry are working to raise their fish more naturally with improved feed, better waste management systems, and other environmental protections. If you choose to eat farmed-fish, try to find quality sources with minimal environmental impact.

Some may be wary of fish after negative health and environmental reports, but fish have many nutritional benefits and are worth including in our diets. Quality sources of fish with low levels of contaminants and not threatened by over-fishing are still available. Find, eat, and enjoy!

Shifting: If your exposure to fish is limited to fish sticks from the frozen food aisle, become familiar with the "Most and Least Desirable" fish list (p.82). Browse the fish case at your grocery store to find what is available and start asking questions. Where is the fish from? When did it come in? Learn the names of fish, how they look, and what they cost. Explain that you would like a safe, clean fish to prepare for your family. Ask for recommendations and cooking suggestions.

A fish market or large health food store may be an even better option. Such stores are used to questions and the staff are usually informed and knowledgeable. Start with a simple white fish fillet to bake, poach, or sauté. In the summer, look for fresh, wild Alaskan or Pacific salmon. Cook steaks, a fillet, or try shellfish in a stir-fry. Stock up on quality frozen fish at the health food store or find online and mail-order resources. Many fish are now Individually Quick Frozen (IQF), or flash frozen, right on the fishing boats after they are caught. This allows you to have quality fish without the pressure of preparing it within 24 hours.

Canned fish (tuna, crab, salmon, and sardines) is also an option. I confess our canned tuna consumption has declined recently, replaced with canned chicken. Read the labels of processed, frozen fish products and avoid those with undesirable additives. Finding quality fish can be expensive and difficult. It can be frustrating to deal with these issues and tempting to avoid fish altogether, but the issues are here to stay. If we learn about them, we can improve and regain one of our most precious, nutritious resources.

Storing: It is best to buy and eat fresh fish with 24 hours or freeze it. Fish should look clear-eyed (if they still have eyes), shiny, and have no "fishy" odor. Thaw frozen fish overnight in the refrigerator and cook it to a temperature of at least 145 degrees.

Shifting Summary

Start with:

- *becoming aware of "Most and Least Desirable" fish (p. 82)*
- *visiting grocery store fish departments, local markets, or health food stores; browse and ask questions*
- *learning to cook a quality white fillet; baking, poaching or sautéing*

Shift to:

- *finding reputable vendors for quality, fresh fish*
- *becoming aware of over-fished species; find alternatives*
- *finding and preparing quality salmon; grilling, broiling, or baking*

Most nutritious:

- *seafood in a stir-fry or soup*
- *becoming aware of fish which are farmed destructively; look for quality farm-raised fish; support the new sustainable aquaculture industry*
- *checking area advisories about the safety of consuming locally caught fish*
- *keeping current on research regarding contamination issues; look for ways to help limit or eliminate contaminates in our environment (see Appendix B)*

FIGURING FISH FOR SENSITIVE POPULATIONS		
Most Desirable (safe to eat 2-3 x/week)	Moderately Desirable (limit to 1x/month)	Least Desirable (avoid)
Anchovies	Blue crab (Gulf	King mackerel
Crab	Coast)	Shark
Flounder (Pacific)	Blue mussels	Swordfish
Herring	Cod (Pacific)	Tilefish (golden
Salmon (Pacific)	Eastern oyster	snapper)
Salmon (wild	Halibut (Alaskan)	Tuna, Bluefin (steaks)
Alaskan)	Lobster	Tuna (canned,
Sardines	Mahi Mahi	albacore)
Sole (Pacific)	Pollock	
Squid	Salmon (Great Lakes)	**Also:**
	Scallops	Halibut (Atlantic)*
Farmed:	Tuna (canned, light)	Largemouth bass
Catfish		Marlin
Clams	**Farmed:**	Oyster (Gulf Coast)
Striped bass	Mussels	Pike
Sturgeon	Oysters	Salmon (Atlantic,
Tilapia		farmed)
Trout		Sea bass
		Walleye
Chilean sea bass*		White croaker
Cod* (Atlantic)		
Flounder* (Atlantic)		
Haddock*		
Orange roughy*		
Shrimp*		
Snapper*		
Sole* (Atlantic)		

Table 18 : Fish for Sensitive Populations
* over-fished or farmed destructively

Local fish from fresh waters also can be contaminated. Check the EPA's regional fish advisories at www.epa.gov/ost/fish.
See Appendix B for more information.

FISH	
What to Limit or Eliminate:	

What to Limit or Eliminate:
Contaminated fish: large, predator (mercury), farmed salmon (POPs)
   shoreline and bottom-feeders near polluted, urban areas
Depleted species or those farmed destructively
Raw or undercooked fish (less than 145 degrees for 15 seconds)
Old fish with cloudy eyes, slimy scales, or "fishy" smell

What to Add or Increase:
Fish from clean waters (especially those high in omega-3 fatty acids)
Individually quick frozen (IQF) or flash-frozen fish from clean waters
Fish canned in water or natural juices; smoked without nitrites

Fish	Description and Uses
Farmed Catfish Tilapia	Also abalone, carp, trout, striped bass, and sturgeon; farmed may contain fewer contaminants; smaller, flat fish (fillet); bake, poach, steam, sauté, or pan-grill
Large Predator* Swordfish Tilefish	Also shark, king mackerel, tilefish, and tuna; deep ocean fish; highest levels of mercury; grill or broil steaks; also marlin and Mahi Mahi
Salmon Wild Alaskan	High omega-3 fatty acids (baking and poaching help preserve omega-3s) king, silver, and sockeye; also Pacific and Atlantic (farmed); grill or broil steaks; bake, poach, steam, sauté, or pan-grill
Sardines	Small, oily fish; high in omega-3 fatty acids; also anchovies and herring; contain bones, good source of calcium; bake, poach, steam, sauté, or pan-grill
Shellfish	Filter-feeders, buy from certified clean areas
Crustaceans	Crab, crawfish, lobster, shrimp; steam, boil, grill, stir-fry, or roast
Mollusks	Clam, mussel, oyster, scallop; steam, sauté, or use in soups and chowders
Cephalopods	Octopus, squid; poach, sauté, broil, or stew
Whitefish	Best to buy offshore, not coastal; Atlantic species are overfished; sole and flounder, mild; cod, haddock, and pollock; also halibut and sea bass, more oily and flavorful; poach, bake, sauté, steam, pan-sear, broil, grill, or roast

Tips:
Always rinse fish with cold water before use
For a "quick thaw," place fish in sealed bag in cold water in refrigerator
How to Store:
Fish: cook same day or freeze (up to three months for oily fish; six months for lean)
Always thaw fish in refrigerator
Canned: up to one year; once open, three to five days in tightly sealed container in refrigerator
Smoked: two to three weeks in the refrigerator

Table 19 : Fish

*may contain high levels of mercury: sensitive populations should avoid

Poultry and Eggs

*"Considering the optimum conditions producers of naturally
raised poultry allow their flocks, antibiotics would rarely
be needed in the first place."*
—Margaret M. Wittenberg, *Good Food*

Poultry refers to chicken, turkey, duck, goose, and other game birds. In the U.S., poultry has become a popular protein choice. We consume mostly chicken and turkey, and eggs from hens. Over the past decade, however, poultry and egg production has shifted dramatically toward factory farming. Egg producers have declined from more than 2,000 in 1990 to less than 300 today. This has a significant impact on the nutritional value of the birds and eggs and poses serious questions about the humane treatment of farm animals.

Benefits: Poultry is a quality source of protein containing all the essential amino acids. Pastured poultry is the most nutrient dense. Birds allowed to forage on grasses contain more omega-3 fatty acids, vitamin A, vitamin E, folic acid, and carotenoids than grain-fed birds.

Eggs are a quick and concentrated source of high-quality protein and contain choline, riboflavin (B2), selenium, iron, folate, vitamins A, B12, D, as well as other trace nutrients. Eggs from pastured poultry will contain less fat, more vitamin A, up to 400 percent more omega-3 fatty acids, and less cholesterol (something poultry scientists have been trying to accomplish for decades). Most of these nutrients, except protein, are found in the yolk. Along with being nutrient-dense, they are easily digested and relatively inexpensive compared to other protein sources.

Issues: The key issues surrounding poultry and eggs are diet and environment. The natural environment for domesticated birds is a combination of shelter and access to the outdoors. Shelter provides fowl protection from predators and a place to roost; while free-roaming allows them to express other natural behaviors such as scratching, pecking, and foraging for grasses, bugs, and other food. As a monogast (having one stomach), chickens are not meant to survive solely on pasture. They obtain up to 30 percent of their diet from grass, clover, and other greens; 50 percent for ducks, geese and other game birds. The rest of their diet needs to be supplemented with grains, legumes, or other sources of high-quality protein.

Chickens can be raised either free range (sometimes called free roaming), cage free (housed but uncaged), or factory farmed. Factory-farmed egg-laying hens are confined in battery cages—stacked wire cages with four birds per cage. Meat birds ("broilers") are housed by the thousands in large warehouses with less than a foot of space per bird. Both types of birds are genetically altered or selectively bred; broilers to grow as large as possible and egg layers to produce as many eggs as possible in the shortest amount of time. This line of thinking may work for efficiency experts on an assembly line but not so well for creating nutrient-dense poultry.

Confined to small spaces and unable to express their natural behaviors, these birds become hostile and peck each other. As a result, the ends of their beaks are clipped off, and, in the case of turkeys, their toes. Meat birds can grow too big and too fast. Their bones can not hold their weight and may develop skeletal problems and deformities. Their lungs and hearts can not keep pace with their bodies, causing a pneumonia-like condition known as ascites. These stresses and unsanitary living conditions can lead to disease, the need for antibiotics and other drugs, and death.

Caged egg layers are subject to constant overhead lighting, fed, and bred to produce the highest quantity of eggs. But chickens, even when supplemented with high amounts of calcium, do not have enough to produce so many egg shells, so it is leached from their bones. This overproduction, coupled with the lack of exercise, causes brittle and broken bones. This condition can lead to paralysis and a potentially fatal disease known as "caged layer fatigue."

Cage-free birds are housed in environments with room to express their natural behaviors such as scratching and roosting but denied access to the outdoors out of concern that extreme weather conditions may negatively impact the birds. They are usually fed a quality vegetarian diet, often organic and supplemented with omega-3 fatty acids. If the birds are labeled "naturally raised," their beaks are not clipped and antibiotics are not used. If birds develop a disease requiring the use of antibiotics, they are sold on the commercial market instead.

Free-range birds have access to open and housed areas. They are free to roam in fenced areas, feeding on bugs, grasses, grains, or legumes. Pastured poultry also has access to grasses, which increase the nutritional content of the birds and their eggs. Opponents argue the uncontrolled diet may include "undesirables" and the varying weather conditions may cause disease. Others feel this is the most natural environment and produces the most nutrient-dense bird.

Eggs have been on a nutritional rollercoaster ever since high cholesterol was linked to heart disease. Although eggs have high dietary cholesterol (found in the yolk), research now demonstrates little correlation between dietary cholesterol and blood cholesterol levels. Those with high blood cholesterol levels, heart disease, or diabetes may need to limit consumption of egg yolks; others can consume an egg or two a day.

The most nutritious eggs are from free-range hens with access to pasture. Cage-free birds fed diets of flax or fish meal also have eggs containing superior nutritional qualities. Eggs from battery-raised birds have the least nutritious eggs and often have a distorted omega-3 and omega-6 fatty acid profile as a result of an all-grain diet. Avoid powdered eggs, which contain oxidized cholesterol.

Salmonella is a bacterial contaminant which can be found in eggs, poultry, meats, and dairy. Previously thought only to exist on the exterior of eggs, research has now shown salmonella can be been found inside a very small percentage of eggs. For this reason, cooking eggs and other animal products thoroughly is recommended, and raw egg consumption is discouraged.

Shifting: Start with looking for cage-free chicken and eggs fed a high-quality vegetarian diet without antibiotics, organic if possible. Poultry raised without a need for antibiotics yields better nutritional quality and is raised under more humane conditions. These products are becoming more available in conventional supermarkets and are easily found in health food stores. Buy boneless breasts and tenders, rinse, marinate, and freeze in portioned bags. They may be more expensive, but they're easier to thaw, prepare, and cook. Try baking or sautéing the chicken and hard boiling or poaching eggs.

Next, search for naturally raised, free-range products. These may not be "organic" as a result of strict labeling standards but generally contain more nutrients than exclusively grain-fed poultry products. Try less-expensive pieces with bones still intact or even a whole bird. Experiment with other types of quality poultry products like ground chicken and turkey, sausages, hot dogs, and lunch meats. Try roasting, grilling, or stir-frying. Make extra for soups, stews, chili, or salads. If cutting back on canned tuna, chicken salad makes a good substitute.

Finally, search for free-range, grass-fed or pastured birds and eggs. Try mail ordering or buy directly from a farm (see Appendix B). Also experiment with other birds such as duck, goose, or game birds. Save the carcass and make your own stock for soups. Maybe even raise your own birds! For nutritional and humane reasons, support growers who produce quality chickens in healthful environments.

Storing: Raw poultry should be cooked within two to three days or frozen. Thaw frozen poultry in the refrigerator and cook thoroughly to an internal temperature of 180-185 degrees or until the juices run clear. Cooked poultry lasts up to four days in the refrigerator. Buy clean, un-cracked, refrigerated eggs. Fresh eggs should be used within four weeks. Keep raw and cooked eggs refrigerated. Do not eat cooked eggs left at room temperature more than two hours, and consider two batches of hard-boiled eggs for Easter egg hunts—one for decorating, hiding, and collecting, and the other for refrigerating and eating.

Shifting Summary

<u>Start with:</u>

- *"naturally-raised" chicken; no antibiotics; bake or stir-fry boneless breasts*
- *cooking eggs thoroughly; boil or poach (less oxidation)*
- *other quality poultry products (ground poultry or sausages)*

<u>Shift to:</u>

- *cage-free birds, organic diet; roast whole bird or parts*
- *finding free-range and/or organic eggs supplemented with flax or fish meal to increase omega-3 fatty acids*
- *trying other quality poultry products (hot dogs or lunch meats)*

<u>Most nutritious:</u>

- *finding local sources for pasture-fed poultry and eggs; visit; buy direct*
- *making stock with leftover poultry products*
- *experimenting with other types of poultry or wild game*

POULTRY and EGGS

What to Limit or Eliminate:

Factory-farmed poultry and eggs; exclusively grain fed
Poultry fed antibiotics and other drugs
Powdered eggs (oxidized cholesterol)

What to Add or Increase:

Cage-free poultry and eggs; organic diet, enhanced with omega-3 fatty
  acids
Free-range poultry and eggs
Pastured poultry and eggs

Poultry	Description and Uses
Birds Chicken Duck Goose Turkey	Birds may be cooked whole, in parts, or ground; for whole birds (trussed or stuffed) roast or bake and use leftovers for broths or soups; for parts (bone-in or boneless, skinless) grill, broil, roast, bake, sauté, or stir-fry; for ground, use like other ground meats: meatloaf, stews, chili, sauces, and other dishes
Bird Products Sausages Hot dogs Deli meats	Look for products without additives such as sodium, MSG, nitrites, refined sweeteners, and artificial colors or flavors; use hot dogs and deli meats individually or on sandwiches; use sausages in soups, stews, sauces, casseroles, or other dishes
Game Birds Guinea hen Partridge Pheasant Quail	Considered "wild," usually farm-raised; cook as you would other poultry*; pheasant — domestic (mild) or wild ("gamy" flavor); quail — small game bird with sweet, tender flavor; also grouse *(*individual differences in birds which may alter cooking instructions)*
Eggs	Hens fed organic diet, flax or fish meal to improve omega-3 fatty acid content; or from cage-free, free-range, or pastured poultry; cook eggs thoroughly (hard-boiled or poached causes less oxidation)

Tips:

Rinse poultry before using; wash hands, utensils thoroughly after handling poultry

Clean cutting boards thoroughly after handling raw poultry (or use separate boards for meats and uncooked foods to avoid possible contamination)

Cook poultry thoroughly (to 180-185 degrees or until juices run clear)

Don't buy or use cracked eggs; wash hands after handling raw eggs

Eggs are a common allergen; vary and rotate them in diet to avoid overexposure

How to Store:

Poultry: use raw poultry within two to four days or freeze

Refrigerate after cooking for up to four days

Eggs: original carton in refrigerator for up to four weeks

Do not leave hard-boiled eggs at room temperature for more than two hours (make two batches at Easter, one for hiding and one for eating)

Table 20 : Poultry and Fish

Dairy

"…dairy products shouldn't occupy the prominent place they do in the USDA food pyramid, nor should they be the centerpiece of the national strategy to prevent osteoporosis. Instead, the evidence shows that dietary calcium should come from a variety of sources… [then] you can look at dairy products as an optional part of a healthy diet and take them in moderation, if at all."
—Walter C. Willett, MD, *Eat Drink, and be Healthy*

Of all the food groups, I found understanding and coming to terms with dairy products the most difficult. Some cultures feel it is unnatural to consume milk from another species. A mammal's milk is specifically designed for their young, and by design, the ability to digest lactose (milk sugar) declines after weaning. Other cultures have consumed dairy products for hundreds of years and have adapted to produce lactase (the enzyme responsible for digesting lactose) into adulthood.

Dairy is a prominent industry in our society and its use often highly debated even within the nutritional field. Our society emphasizes dairy as an important source of calcium. But, surprisingly, cultures with little or no dairy have the strongest teeth and bones. Some Asian cultures take in less than half the recommended daily allowance (RDA) for calcium yet they have the lowest rates of osteoporosis and bone fractures. While our society, with one of the highest intakes of dairy (25 percent of our diet), also has one of the highest rates osteoporosis and bone fractures.* Is dairy consumption unnatural and unhealthful or a sign of genetic evolution?

*The high bone density of cultures with minimal calcium intake may be due to a number of factors: consuming calcium in forms more readily absorbed by the body, a higher intake of alkaline-forming foods, consuming fewer calcium inhibitors such as protein, sugar, and soda, and getting more exercise.

Benefits: Dairy products such as milk, cream, cheese, yogurt, and butter, are made primarily from the milk of cows, but also other mammals such as sheep and goats. They contain varying amounts of protein, fats, carbohydrates, calcium, vitamin A, riboflavin (B2), other B vitamins, phosphorus, magnesium, potassium, and sodium. Cows raised entirely on grass have higher amounts of beta-carotene, vitamin A and E, 500 percent more conjugated linoleic acid (CLA), an important omega-3 fatty acid, and a healthier omega-3 to omega-6 ratio. In fact, the more grain an animal consumes, the more unbalanced the essential fatty acid ratio becomes.

Issues: There are several issues surrounding dairy products: concerns about how animals are raised, how products are processed, digestion difficulties, calcium absorption problems, and saturated fat and cholesterol in butter.

Factory-farmed cows are bred, fed, and injected with hormones* to produce large amounts of milk. Along with diluting nutrients, this overproduction of milk can cause frequent infections (mastitis) requiring the constant use of antibiotics. Concerns about the health impact of hormone use on animals and humans and the development of antibiotic-resistant bacteria have led many to protest a practice unnecessary in the first place. We have an abundance of milk, not a shortage. Animals not stimulated with high-protein diets and hormones to overproduce milk have higher concentrations of nutrients in their products. Quality is better than quantity.

> *The recombinant Bovine Growth Hormone (rBGH) is a genetically engineered synthetic growth hormone used to increase milk production in dairy cows. It was introduced to the market in 1994 by the Monsanto Company and is used on approximately one-third of the cows in the US. Its use is banned in Canada, the European Union has a declared moratorium on the subject due to questions about its impact on human and animal health, and the Codex Commission (the United Nations main food safety body) refused to endorse the safety of rBGH, allowing countries to deny imports of rBGH-treated dairy products. Products containing rBGH do not have to be labeled, so inquiring directly to manufacturers or buying organic is the only way to ensure you are consuming hormone-free dairy products. Products from Canada, New Zealand, and Australia, and countries in the European Union, are also rBGH free. (See Appendix B for further resources.)*

Milk is usually processed in three ways: pasteurized, homogenized, and fortified. During pasteurization, milk is heated to destroy harmful bacteria and enzymes that sour the milk. Homogenization is the process of breaking up fat globules to provide a uniform consistency, and fortification provides synthetic vitamins, such as A and D, which help calcium absorption. While pasteurization is required by law, homogenization is not, but it is typically performed so the cream does not rise to the surface of the milk.

Many in the nutritional community are advocating the return to raw (unpasteurized) dairy products. They state past sanitary concerns leading to the need for pasteurization are no longer relevant and that certified raw milk from healthy, pasture-fed cows is the least processed, most nutritious, and best assimilated product. Pasteurization destroys or denatures enzymes, vitamins, proteins, and beneficial bacteria which help break down lactose (milk sugar) and casein (milk protein) and cause a host of health-related ailments. For this reason, raw milk products and fermented or "cultured" dairy products such as yogurt, buttermilk, cottage cheese, and cheeses with added enzymes are easier to digest and absorb. The availability of certified raw milk varies from state to state. Some states allow it to be sold commercially; in others, it must be bought directly from a farm or cow share program (see Appendix B for resources and more information.)*

> *(Disclaimer): Many health authorities oppose the consumption of unpasteurized milk products for safety reasons and, by executive order, it is forbidden to transport raw milk across state lines.*

Many people, in fact the majority of the world's population, are lactose intolerant (difficulty digesting the milk sugar lactose.) Lactase, an enzyme produced by infants to help digest milk, usually disappears as children mature. This is why many people, especially those of Asian, African, Mediterranean, and Hispanic descent (or anyone whose ancestors did not consume dairy) have difficulty digesting lactose. Other cultures (northern Europeans and their descendants), however, have consumed dairy products for so many generations that their bodies have genetically adjusted to produce lactase into adulthood.

Casein (milk protein) is also difficult to digest and one of the most common food allergens. Many people experiencing dairy-related health problems (cramping, bloating, diarrhea, ear infections, sinus problems, and other mucous-related health issues) are unaware of the food-ailment connection. Eliminating dairy products for one to two weeks (not an easy task for most Americans whose diet is 25 percent dairy products) may alleviate many symptoms. Others have found goat milk, which has a fatty acid and protein structure different from cow milk, easier to digest. Experiment or seek guidance from a nutrition expert (see Appendix C).

Consuming dairy products is often equated with obtaining calcium. But ingesting calcium is different from absorbing and utilizing calcium. For the body to absorb and utilize calcium, it requires the proper balance of other nutrients, mainly magnesium, as well as a low intake of calcium inhibitors. The typical American diet is high in acid-producing foods such as coffee, colas, refined flour, and animal protein; and low in alkaline-producing foods like vegetables. To help maintain the proper acid /alkaline balance for the body's internal environment, calcium and other alkalinizing minerals are leached from the bones to neutralize the acid. Over time, this can lead to depletion of calcium reserves and bone thinning. (For more information see Appendix B).

Magnesium plays a major role in the absorption and proper utilization of calcium as well as other nutrients. Magnesium absorption and utilization is inhibited by several factors: diets high in phosphorus* (found in animal protein, milk, and cola products) and sugar cause magnesium to be excreted from the body. Too much calcium, absorbed by the same part of the intestines, can also block magnesium absorption.

Dairy products are high in calcium but low in magnesium. Milk also has a one-to-one calcium-to-phosphorus ratio, which interferes with calcium absorption. Whole grains, dark leafy greens, and beans contain calcium and magnesium as well as other nutrients which help move calcium into the bones. This is why Americans, despite having one of the highest calcium intakes in the world, also have one the highest rates of osteoporosis and bone fractures. It is important to get enough calcium, and make sure you have an adequate supply of magnesium to help absorb and properly metabolize calcium into your bones. Nan Kathryn Fuchs, PhD states in the *User's Guide to Calcium and Magnesium*, "When it comes to calcium and magnesium, you are not what you eat. You are what you eat, digest, and absorb."

> *The phosphoric acid, prominent in most cola drinks, is particularly problematic for teenagers. At a time of increased bone growth when calcium absorption is essential, many teenagers are switching from milk to soda and leaching more calcium from the body. Compounding the problem are cash-tight schools using vending machines to help supplement budgets and advertisers capitalizing on adolescents' vulnerability to peers and outside influences.*

Butter is made from the cream, or fat, of churned milk. It contains fat-soluble vitamins A, D, K, and E as well as essential fatty acids and trace minerals such as the antioxidant selenium. The body uses natural saturated fats as an important source of energy and nutrients as well as to cushion vital organs. Butter, like eggs, contains lecithin, which helps break down and metabolize cholesterol.

Butter has been banished from many households because it is high in saturated fat and cholesterol. Unfortunately, it is often replaced with less desirable processed products and unstable oils for cooking. Butter, however, is a whole food rich with nutrients that cultures have been consuming for generations well before heart disease made itself known. While it is important to limit consumption of saturated fats, butter is a better and more nutritious choice than shortening and margarine, which contain trans-fatty acids, and it is a more stable fat than plant oils for high-heat cooking.

For those who can tolerate dairy products, quality sources can provide nutrients and be part of a varied diet. For those who prefer not to consume dairy products, have a lactose intolerance, or are allergic, calcium can easily be obtained and absorbed from other food sources or from properly balanced calcium supplements.

Shifting: My use of dairy has come full circle. I used to consume large amounts of dairy, especially while pregnant to help control gestational diabetes. I should not have been surprised when this child was born with a milk allergy. Dairy products, once a staple in our refrigerator, went out and panic set in. "Got milk?" No, I didn't. I was conditioned to think dairy products were essential and felt we had a gaping hole in our diets. After finding alternative sources of nutrients and calcium, I am more comfortable about meeting my family's dietary needs (although not totally relaxed since I use a calcium supplement, just in case.)

Now we are beginning to include moderate amounts of dairy products again. We use them like condiments—raw milk cheese on a sandwich, yogurt in a smoothie, and, of course, a little ice cream. My daughter seems to tolerate small amounts and will eventually have to make her own decisions about what to include in her diet and how it makes her feel. Our other calcium/magnesium-rich sources include almond butter, beans, seeds, dark leafy greens, (I even put seaweed in soups but don't tell my family) as well as that little calcium supplement, just in case.

In the very least, switch to hormone-free and antibiotic-free dairy products. Organic products are becoming readily available in most supermarkets. Some may even have pasteurized milk that has not been homogenized. Avoid "ultra-pasteurized" and "imitation" products, those with additives, and processed cheeses. Yogurt, raw milk cheeses, and other cultured or fermented products may be easier to digest. Use butter instead of margarine. For those who are cholesterol sensitive or concerned about saturated fats, olive oil can be a satisfying replacement for butter. It can be used on vegetables and even toast. Another popular modification is to make a "better butter" by mixing half softened butter with half olive oil in a food processor until blended and storing it in the refrigerator. Use it as a spread in place of butter.

Next, search for products from grass-fed animals which contain more nutrients, and research raw milk products (see Appendix B). Finally, if you think you may be experiencing milk-related health problems, consider abstaining for a few weeks or seek nutritional advice (see Appendix C).

Storing: To obtain maximum freshness, keep dairy products refrigerated and out of direct light. Follow "use by" dates labeled on packages. Hard cheeses last longer than soft. Butter and some cheeses may be frozen to extend shelf life.

Shifting Summary

Start with:
- *dairy products free of hormones and antibiotics*
- *butter instead of margarine or vegetable shortening*
- *cutting back on calcium inhibitors (phosphorus, soda, sugar, and excess animal protein)*

Shift to:
- *organic dairy products*
- *removing dairy for two weeks if concerned about dairy consumption; or try goat milk and goat milk products*
- *looking for other sources of calcium and magnesium (whole grains, leafy greens, beans, nuts, seeds, or even sea "vegetables")*

Most nutritious:
- *100 percent grass-fed dairy products*
- *investigating raw milk and finding local resources*
- *researching natural food cooperatives, buying clubs, mail order, or local sources for organic and/or grass-fed products*

DAIRY
What to Limit or Eliminate:
Dairy products that use bovine growth hormones (rBGH) and antibiotics
Dairy products with artificial additives, colorings, flavorings, and refined sweeteners
Powdered milk (oxidized cholesterol) and processed cheeses
Margarine and vegetable shortening
What to Add or Increase:
Dairy products free of hormones and antibiotics or organic
Fermented or cultured dairy products
Dairy products from grass-fed animals
Butter and clarified butter (ghee)

Dairy	Description and Uses
Butter	Churned cream; at least 80 percent fat; also clarified butter (ghee), free of lactose and casein and able to withstand higher temperatures for cooking
Cheese	Protein, calcium, phosphorus, vitamin A, fat, and sodium;
Hard	Good for grating; Parmesan, Romano
Semifirm	Good for melting; cheddar, Swiss
Soft-ripened	White crust, smooth inside; Brie, Camembert
Semisoft	Firmer than soft ripened; Havarti, Provolone
Blue-veined	Inoculated with mold; Roquefort, Stilton, Gorgonzola
Cottage cheese	Cultured curds mixed with cream and salt
Cream	Fat from whole milk; available in light and heavy (used for whipping); half-and-half is a mixture of milk and cream; also sour cream (cultured)
Cream Cheese	Cultured cream; high in fat and cholesterol
Ice cream	Made from 10 percent or more milk fat; look for all-natural
Milk	Available skim, low-fat, flavored
Certified Raw	Unpasteurized; available in some states
Goat	Fatty acid and protein structure different from cow milk; more easily digested
Buttermilk	Cultured or "soured;" more easily digested

Yogurt	Fermented milk; look for "active yogurt cultures" (bacteria) and natural sweeteners; use with and after antibiotics to help replenish important intestinal bacteria; also kefir, a milk-based cultured drink similar to yogurt

Tips:

Yogurt or kefir with "active cultures" helps replace beneficial intestinal bacteria during and after antibiotic use

Do not give whole milk to a baby under one year of age (interferes with iron absorption)

Healthier butter: make your own spread by mixing half olive oil with half butter; store in container in refrigerator

How to Store:

In refrigerator out of light in closed containers

Hard cheese: several weeks in refrigerator; soft cheeses: several days in refrigerator

Table 21 : Dairy

High Calcium Sources	High Magnesium Sources	Calcium Inhibitors
Dried seaweeds (hijiki, wakame, kelp, Kombu)	Dried seaweeds (wakame, kombu, kelp, hijiki, arame)	Coffee and soft drinks
Hard cheeses (Parmesan, Romano)	Beans (soy, mung, aduki, black)	Excess animal protein
Wheat grass, barley grass	Whole Grains (buckwheat, millet, wheat berries, corn)	High phosphorus
Sardines	Nuts (almonds, cashews, filberts)	Lack of exercise
Almonds	Seeds (sesame)	Sugar
Amaranth (grain)	High-chlorophyll foods (green plants, wheat grass, barley grass, microalgae such as spirulina, and chlorella)	
Greens* (collards, kale, turnip)		
Quinoa (grain)		
Tofu		
Milk		
Beans (black, pinto, garbanzo)		
Yogurt		
Seeds (sunflower, sesame)		
Nuts (Brazil, walnuts)		
Figs		
Sardines		
Salmon (canned)		

*Most green plants provide balanced sources of calcium and other cofactors which help increase absorption and utilization. Spinach, chard, and beet greens, however, contain oxalic acid which interferes with absorption.

**Presoak grains and legumes to help neutralize phytic acid which can bind with calcium and other minerals interfering with absorption

Meats

"Despite all the grim, dismal facts about modern meat production, eating meat is still a fundamentally healthy thing to do, provided the meat is grown naturally, is handled in a sanitary manner, and is part of a balanced whole-food diet."
—Chris Kilham, *The Whole Food Bible*

Meat is not the problem; it is meat as we know it today. The meat available in the grocery stores is a far cry from what used to be a healthful part of our ancestors' diet. They ate meat but had fewer heart attacks, cancers, and other meat-related health issues. So, what is the difference?

Benefits: Meat is most commonly equated with beef, but also includes pork, lamb, and other "game" meats such as bison, deer, rabbit, and buffalo. Meat is a concentrated source of protein, iron, zinc, selenium, phosphorus, and B vitamins. Pasture-raised beef, lamb, and pork contains less fat, fewer calories, more vitamin E, and is higher in omega-3 fatty acids. Grass-fed beef products also have more beta-carotene, a better omega-3 to omega-6 fatty acid ratio than grain-fed animals, and higher amounts of conjugated linoleic acid (CLA), an important essential fatty acid. In fact, ruminants (animals with multi-chambered stomachs such as cattle, sheep, goats, bison, and deer) which thrive grazing on pasture, have two to five times more CLA.

Issues: Concerns about meat center on how animals are raised and fed, safe handling and processing procedures, and the fat and cholesterol content. Today, most animals raised for meat are transferred to large feedlots where they are confined in crowded, unsanitary conditions and fed grains, animal byproducts, and other questionable material (trash and manure.) They are bred, fed, injected with hormones, and treated with low-level antibiotics for the sole purpose of getting them to market as quickly as possible. These conditions lead to sickness, stress, disease, and the need for more antibiotics and other drugs.*

> *More than half the antibiotics produced each year in the U.S. are used on factory-farmed livestock to promote growth and keep germs at bay. When illnesses occur, as they often do in overcrowded, unsanitary conditions, more antibiotics are used. This is fostering the development of drug-resistant offspring and strains of "super germs." As a result, antibiotic- resistant bacteria are "rendering most of our important antibiotics ineffective."*

Grain is not the natural diet of ruminants and certainly not animal by-products, trash, and manure. Grains fatten animals quickly while the questionable feed is inexpensive, but these foods stress the animals' systems and provide inadequate nutrients. Animals can become sick or die; with the use of animal by-products, we may become sick or die. The threat of "mad cow" disease has sent the hardiest meat-eater running for the hills of vegetarianism. "Without announcing the fact, feedlot managers had been turning herbivores into cannibals, violating a natural barrier that had protected them from disease," states Jo Robinson, author of *Pasture Perfect.* "What's more, this is not just another case of good meat being contaminated with bacteria; the meat itself was bad. No amount of hand washing or knife cleaning or cooking was going to get rid of the problem."*

> *Mad-cow disease is a transmissible spongiform encephalopathy (TSE), a fatal brain disease called Creutzfeldt-Jakob disease in humans, scrapie in sheep, and chronic wasting disease in deer and elk. It is believed mutant proteins, or prions, are acquired by consuming infected animals. To reduce risk, avoid eating brains and processed beef products such as ground meat, hot dogs, and sausages, or purchase organic or 100 percent grass-fed beef, which are not fed animal remains. Those with low risk tolerance may choose to avoid products altogether until more information is known.*

High-speed slaughtering and processing procedures in unsanitary conditions has led to contaminated meat products. Bacteria such as Salmonella, Listeria, and E. coli are spread due to pressure to maintain maximum productivity schedules and keep costs down. While some companies have implemented their own strict quality control procedures (HACCP,*) others still look to debatable technologies such as irradiation to override problems rather than solve them. Bacteria on whole meats can be killed by properly cooking the surface of meats. Ground meats, however, such as sausages and hamburgers, which may use the parts of various animals and mix them, need to be cooked thoroughly. Suggestions are provided by the Food Safety and Inspection Service at www. fsis.usda.gov/OA/pubs/facts_basics.htm. As with fish, be familiar with meat growers and processors. Find products that are free of hormones and antibiotics, and processed under safe, sanitary conditions.

> ** The Food and Drug Administration (FDA) is in the process of implementing a new system to help prevent hazards that could cause food-borne illnesses. Hazard Analysis and Critical Point Control, or HACCP (pronounced "hassip"), uses science-based controls to follow foods such as seafood and juice from raw material to finished product. Pilot programs have begun for dairy, while some in the meat and poultry industry voluntarily apply HACCP procedures (the USDA regulates meat and poultry.) For more information see* www. cfsan.fda.gov/~lrd/haccp.html.

Meats had been nourishing cultures for thousands of years before the onset of so much heart disease and high cholesterol. However, current methods of feeding animals grain do produce meats high in saturated fats, cholesterol, and omega-6 fatty acids, and low in omega-3 fatty acids and CLA. Diets high in saturated fats have been linked to heart disease. If you do choose to consume grain-fed meats, trimming excess fat (this also reduces toxins), eating smaller portions, and limiting frequency of consumption can help make meat part of healthful diet. Responding to our society's desire for leaner meat, beef producers are trying to genetically breed leaner cows, slaughter them earlier, and trim excess fat. This same goal is accomplished by feeding animals grass. This takes time and space however, and works against the "bigger, better, faster" mentality.

Most of the issues surrounding meats can be solved by returning animals to their natural diet and environment of pasture. They are a healthful source of nutrients, but additional planning and management may be required. Grass-fed meats take longer to produce, may be harder to find, more expensive, and, being leaner, need to be cooked properly. If you eat choose to eat meat, make an effort to find products raised in humane conditions, free of antibiotics and hormones, which have been handled and processed properly.

Shifting: Consuming enough meat is not a problem for most people in the U.S. In fact, most could benefit from reducing and re-placing meat with other quality sources of protein (beans, fish, eggs, nuts, seeds, and some whole grains) and other nutrient-dense foods. By increasing other inexpensive healthful foods, meat consumption will naturally decrease, making quality meat products more affordable. Portions of meat from a typical meal can last for two or three meals.

Start by searching the regular supermarket for hormone-free and antibiotic-free meat products. Organic, grain-fed meats are also an option but not as nutrient-dense as grass-fed. Look for lean cuts of meat, trim excess fat, and cook properly. Prepared meat products such as hot dogs, lunch meats, and sausages often contain undesirable additives such as the preservatives BHT and BHA, the curing agent sodium nitrite,* and flavorings made from refined sugars. Search for more healthful, more natural forms of these products.

---

* When meats containing nitrites, such as bacon, sausage, and ham, are heated to high temperatures, they form nitrosamine, a potent carcinogenic compound. Some cured meats are available without nitrites. They are usually found in the frozen food section, need to be thawed in the refrigerator, and should be used within four to five days.

Next, start investigating grass-fed products. Search health food stores, mail order, or online. Look for products labeled "pasture-finished," "grass-finished," or "100 percent grass-fed." "Pasture-raised" is also an option and means animals may have been supplemented with non-grass products when high-quality grass was unavailable. Compare prices and shipping costs (many suppliers will not ship during the summer.) They may be expensive and hard to find now, but with more demand, the market will respond. Become familiar with meat processing procedures and support companies with high-quality, safe, sanitary conditions.

Finally, if you are fortunate to have a local supplier in your area, visit, ask questions, and find out how the animals are raised. (If they don't offer a tour, don't buy.) Many community farms offer produce, dairy, and meat. Start slowly and move on to other food products as you become comfortable. Also, consider your storage capabilities for large quantities of frozen meat products. Other game meats are becoming popular and available, so try them if you are feeling adventurous. Give your meat-eating teeth a little practice.

Storing: Meat can become contaminated with bacteria. Handle and cook meat properly to eliminate the risk of contracting a food-borne illness. Keep raw meat and its juices separate from ready-to-eat foods. Wash hands, utensils, and cutting boards thoroughly after handling raw meats, and make sure meats are cooked and stored properly.

Shifting Summary

Start with:
- *hormone-free and antibiotic-free products; other meat products without additives*
- *trimming excess fat; cutting portion size and frequency*
- *cooking ground meat thoroughly*

Shift to:
- *searching health food stores, farmers' markets, and online for grass-fed products*
- *organic or "pasture-raised" products*
- *other protein sources (beans, fish, and eggs)*

Most nutritious:
- *searching for grass-fed animal products in stores, mail-order, online, or*

through buyer's clubs; compare prices; evaluate storage options
• *considering local grass-fed animal products; visit and ask questions*
• *experimenting with other game meats*

MEATS	
What to Limit or Eliminate: Meat from animals fed grains and other questionable feed Meat from animals given antibiotics and hormones Poorly processed and poorly prepared meats Large amounts of saturated fats	
What to Add or Increase: Meats free of antibiotics or hormones; safely handled, safely processed meats Organic meats and/or pasture-fed animal products Lean meats	
Meats	**Description and Uses**
Beef	Graded by Prime, Choice, Select; cubes, strips, tips; sauté, stir-fry, or kebabs
Chuck	neck, shoulder, blade; roast or stew
Rib	rib or rib-eye; roast, sauté, broil, or grill*
Loin	shell, tenderloin; roast, sauté, broil, or grill*
Flank	under the loin; sauté, broil, pan-grill, or grill*
Sirloin	behind flank, loin; roast, sauté, broil, or grill* steaks
Round	ground meat; use for burgers or stir-fry
Pork	
Shoulder	Rump; also picnic shoulder; roast
Loin	pork chops, tenderloins; roast or sauté
Belly	ribs (parboil, grill); bacon (fry)
Leg	ham; usually cured (see "Cured Meats")
Lamb	Leg, chops, rack, loin (more tender); roast, broil, sauté, or grill (dry-heat cooking) shoulder, shank, breast (less-tender cuts); stew or braise
Cured -Meats	
Bacon	Pork belly; cured in brine, smoked
Ham	Cooked, sliced (deli)
Luncheon	May be cured or uncured
Sausage	Meat, fat, spices

Game	Venison, buffalo, rabbit, and other wild animals

Tips:
Reduce frequency and portion size; make meat a side dish rather than center of a meal
For tough cuts of meat, try slow cooker and pressure cooker
Wash hands thoroughly with hot soapy water before and after handling raw meat
Keep all utensils and cutting boards for raw meat separate and wash thoroughly

How to Store:
Use "sell by" date or freeze up to three months
Defrost in refrigerator
Refrigerate leftovers quickly; use within three to four days or freeze

Table 22 : Meat

*The nitrites and nitrates in meats can form carcinogens when grilled or fried.

Condiments, Flavorings, and Supplements

Condiments: As with other foods, look for products made with real ingredients. Syrups, salad dressings, ketchups, and other condiments are notorious for added sugar and other highly refined additives. Read labels, buy quality condiments, and make what you can at home: salsas, salad dressings, marinades are best fresh, so develop your own special recipes.

Herbs and Spices: Buy and learn how to use quality herbs and spices. Dried herbs are more concentrated than fresh herbs; one tablespoon of fresh herbs equals one teaspoon of dry. Basil, cilantro, oregano, parsley, rosemary, and thyme are popular in soups, salads, and sauces or to season fish, poultry and meats. Sweet spices such as cinnamon and nutmeg are great in baked goods, desserts, warm breakfast cereals, and smoothies. Choose chili powder or cumin for spicier, hot dishes with a Mexican flavor.

Supplements: Although the basic premise of supplements (ingesting isolated substances such as vitamins, minerals, protein powders, or "green food") seems to go against the concept of whole foods, supplementation can be beneficial or even necessary. A history of poor eating habits or individual health problems may require extra resources to balance body chemistry or counteract health limitations. Those deficient in a particular nutrient may benefit from taking vitamin or mineral supplements; protein powders may help someone with blood sugar issues; and products containing chlorophyll can help cleanse the body of toxins. Others may use supplements to obtain optimal rather than merely adequate nutrition.

But simply taking vitamins and supplements cannot make up for a poor diet, especially with conventional vitamins. As with real foods, processing can harm the nutrients, and care needs to be taken to preserve the quality of supplements. Many mass-produced products are processed at high heat, damaging or destroying the nutrients, while others have added colors, fillers, coatings, and poor-quality ingredients. If you choose to supplement your diet, find quality sources and proper guidance about amounts, effects, and interactions (see Appendix C). Ideally, by eating a nutritious, real-foods diet from the beginning, we would not need supplementation—a goal our children can aspire to.

Shifting Strategies Summary

Start with:

Whole Grains:
- brown rice, rolled oats, and more "whole"-some grain products
- unbleached white flour for baking; replace one quarter to one-third with whole wheat flour
- whole grains and whole-grain products available in regular supermarket

Vegetables and Fruits
- fresh vegetables and salad daily with dinner; use leftovers in eggs or for lunch
- dried fruit for snacks; make smoothies; vegetable snacks with dips
- vegetable breads, muffins, and pancakes (use extra pumpkin puree in pancake batter); stock up on quality frozen produce (canned, if necessary)

Nuts, Seeds, and Oils
- replacing rancid nuts and seeds; use fresh for snacks, salads, and baked goods
- replacing refined "vegetable" and hydrogenated oils (margarine and shortening)
- finding a quality brand of peanut butter, free of sugars and hydrogenated oil

Legumes:
- canned beans: rinsed, sprinkled on salads (chick peas or kidney beans)
- using baked or refried beans as a side dish
- making chili, burritos, or other beans meals; using canned beans in soup

Sweeteners
- quality brands of jam, honey, and pure maple syrup
- natural sugar and reduced amounts in baking

- removing highly refined and artificial sweeteners (especially sodas)

Fish

- becoming aware of "Most and Least Desirable" fish (p. 83)
- visiting grocery store fish departments, local markets, or health food stores; browse and ask questions
- learning to cook a quality white fillet; baking, poaching or sautéing

Poultry and Eggs

- "naturally-raised" chicken; no antibiotics; bake or stir-fry boneless breasts
- cooking eggs thoroughly; boil or poach (less oxidation)
- other quality poultry products (ground poultry or sausages)

Dairy

- dairy products free of hormones and antibiotics
- butter instead of margarine or vegetable shortening
- cutting back on calcium inhibitors (phosphorus, soda, sugar, and excess animal protein)

Meat

- hormone-free and antibiotic-free products; other meat products without additives
- trimming excess fat; cutting portion size and frequency
- cooking ground meat thoroughly

Shift to:

Whole Grains

- steel-cut oats or other multi-grain hot cereals; other whole grain flours
- pre-cooking whole grains (barley, millet, or quinoa); add to a soup, salad, pilaf, or as a side dish
- sprouted grain bread products; pairing grains and beans at meals

Vegetables and Fruits

- various vegetable families; serve dark leafy greens once a week
- soup once or twice a month; stew, chili, or slow-cooker recipes with fresh produce
- learning basic vegetable stir-fry, casserole, and pasta recipes
- MYOM with fresh, quality produce (pizzas and Mexican dishes)

Nuts, Seeds, and Oils

- new nut butters for sandwiches, snacks, dipping, or in smoothies
- quality olive and sesame oil for dressings and low-temperature cooking
- butter or coconut oil for medium to high heat

Legumes:

- lentil or split pea soups (no soaking required)
- bean spreads and dips: hummus or white bean
- tofu in a smoothie or stir-fry

Sweeteners

- natural, sweet spices and flavorings like cinnamon, nutmeg, and vanilla
- reading labels for hidden sugars; buying better-quality products
- baking with reduced amounts of sugar; including other nutrient-dense ingredients

Fish

- finding reputable vendors for quality, fresh fish
- becoming aware of overfished species; find alternatives
- finding and preparing quality salmon; grill, broil, or bake

Poultry and Eggs

- cage-free birds, organic diet; roast whole bird or parts
- finding free-range and/or organic eggs; supplemented with flax or fish meal to increase omega-3 fatty acids
- trying other quality poultry products (hot dogs or lunch meats)

Dairy

- organic dairy products
- removing dairy for two weeks if concerned about dairy consumption

- looking for other sources of calcium and magnesium (whole grains, leafy greens, beans, nuts, seeds, or even sea "vegetables")

Meat

- searching health food store, farmers' markets, and online for grass-fed products
- organic and "pasture-raised" products
- other protein sources (beans, fish, and eggs)

Most Nutritious:

Whole Grains

- visiting health food stores for (organic) whole grains and whole-grain flours
- soaking, sprouting, and grinding your own grains
- researching natural food cooperatives, buying clubs, and mail-order grain products

Vegetables and Fruits

- buying a juicer and learn how to juice produce
- starting a garden or joining a community farm (CSA)
- researching natural food cooperatives, buying clubs, and mail-order organic products

Nuts, Seeds, and Oils

- flax seed oil on salads, pasta, toast, or oatmeal; keep refrigerated
- finding a source for organic nuts, seeds, and oils (health food stores, food co-ops, mail)
- grinding fresh nut butters; soaking and/or sprouting nuts and seeds

Legumes

- soaking dried beans and cooking; try a three-bean salad, rice and beans, or casserole
- experimenting with other soy products: miso, tempeh, tamari, and natto
- finding resources for quality, organic legumes

Sweeteners

- experimenting with other natural sweeteners; switch, reduce, remove

- reading informational material about the negative effects of sugar (see Appendix B)
- visiting the health food store for greater variety of natural and organic sweeteners

Fish

- seafood in a stir-fry or soup
- becoming aware of fish which are farmed destructively; look for quality farm-raised fish; support the new sustainable aquaculture industry
- checking area advisories about the safety of consuming locally caught fish
- keeping current on research regarding contamination issues; look for ways to help limit or eliminate contaminates in our environment (see Appendix B)

Poultry and Eggs

- finding local sources for pasture-fed poultry and eggs; visit; buy direct
- making stock with leftover poultry products
- experimenting with other types of poultry or wild game

Dairy

- 100 percent grass-fed dairy products
- investigating information on raw milk and find local resources
- researching natural food cooperatives, buying clubs, mail order, or local sources for organic and/or grass-fed products

Meat

- searching for grass-fed animal products in stores, mail-order, online, or through buyers' clubs; compare prices; evaluate storage options
- considering local grass-fed animal products; visit and ask questions
- experimenting with other game meats

Real Foods Summary

There are better, more healthful, and more humane ways to produce foods than agribusiness and factory farming. Look for sustainable farming methods which preserve nutrients, the environment, animal welfare, and human health at the same time.

Take time to evaluate the foods you eat on a regular basis. What foods do you want more of? Which foods do you want less of? Shift the balance. You may want to decrease refined grain products, dairy, and meats, and increase whole grains, vegetables, and beans. Use *The Shifting Strategies Summary*, in the previous section to help guide your transition.

It is hard to change habits which have been ingrained for years. Many do not know anything else. Unlearning and relearning a new way to do something requires effort and persistence. But it will become easier and more enjoyable—this from someone who used the same small bottle of dish soap for an entire year (still half full.) I ate frozen dinners every night and washed one fork. I had a very clean kitchen but a very unhealthy body. Now my kitchen is a mess and I feel great. Relax, savor the flavors, and enjoy the tastes of real foods.

Feeding the Family

"I was a wonderful parent—until I had children."
—Adele Faber, *How to Talk So Kids Will Listen*

Introduction

We can now define, find, and fix healthful food; but how do we get children to eat it? Getting children to eat well seems to be more about parenting skills than nutritious food. Before I had children, I envisioned us in our aprons cooking away in the kitchen. When they arrived, my visions were replaced with hungry, whining children attached to my legs as I shuffled around trying to get dinner ready. I thought we would shop together, read labels, and pick fresh foods. Now I am lucky to come home with the items on my list. Pleasant meals gave way to pleas, bribes, and battles to eat particular foods. But I want my children to be healthy and well fed. So how do I get them to want to eat nutritious food?

I struggled with this question for some time. I read, talked with people, gathered ideas, tips, tricks, and rules. Then I realized I had learned this lesson before: trust the intelligence of the body. We are all born with internal hunger cues. We become hungry, we eat. The key is to work with these natural hunger cues and to guide children to acknowledge and satisfy them in healthful ways. When children become hungry, it is the parents' responsibility to provide healthful food. The child decides what to eat and how much.

In the morning, when your child asks for breakfast, responses such as "Oh, you're hungry? What do you feel like eating?" helps them to make intrinsic connections. We eat to satisfy hunger and our bodies can help guide our decisions.* Offer a variety of nutritious food choices and let them eat the amount they want. When they are done, ask if they are full to reinforce the cue to stop eating. Denying or limiting food when children are hungry can create feelings of anxiety and deprivation, causing overcompensation. Bribing and force-feeding children who are full can override the body's natural satiety mechanisms.

> ** This process can become distorted by introducing processed and refined foods which unbalance body chemistry and condition children to unnatural tastes and textures. Children on this path may require extra effort to recondition the body to real foods and rebalance body chemistry. Some children may also have sensory issues (aversions to smells, tastes, or textures) which affect eating habits. Appetite changes can also be a result of anxiety or depression. If you suspect these issues, it may be helpful to seek professional guidance.*

I also guide food choices in other ways. I introduce new and more nutrient-dense foods when children are the most hungry (and hold back "favorites"). If my children "feel like" ice cream for breakfast, I explain ice cream is more of a dessert food and suggest yogurt as a more appropriate breakfast food to start their day. Children need to build a framework for making healthful dietary decisions. Just as we guide children to be active during the day and rest during the night for optimal health, we also guide them to the foods which give them energy, help them grow, and maintain their health.

Children should have pleasant and positive associations with eating. Parents decide what will be available, and children decide if they will eat it and how much. Keep healthful food in the house and have realistic expectations. Other strategies for helping to encourage healthy eating in children are listed below.

Tools for Encouraging Healthy Eating

Modeling: Being a role model is one of the most critical factors in shaping a child's eating habits. What people do speaks louder than what they say. Children are going to want to eat what we eat. If we want children to make healthy choices and respect themselves, we have to demonstrate these qualities in our own lives. Show them how to trust hunger cues. Our bodies tell us when and what to eat. "I'm hungry for a snack. I feel like eating a piece of fruit." If we eat for other reasons (boredom, stress, or depression) or have anxieties about food, children may internalize these messages too. Eat healthful food, enjoy it, and help model the connection between eating well and feeling good.

Experience: Provide opportunities for them to be around healthful food and make healthful food choices. Encourage them to become involved in the process whenever possible from start to finish. They can help plan, buy, prepare, cook, and clean. (See list of Age Appropriate Activities p. 124). The more involved they are in the process, the more invested they will become, and more likely to eat healthful food. These experiences also make for quality time with children. They will feel valued and want to make healthful choices.

Give children control over what to eat whenever possible. Have them choose foods at the grocery store. "We need vegetables for dinner. Which would you like?" Use the same technique at meals and snacks. "Would you like fish or chicken for dinner? What snack do you feel like eating?" As children become older, have them participate in planning meals and preparing shopping lists. Continue to increase experiences, opportunities, and responsibilities as children grow.

Knowledge: Give children information about why we make certain decisions. With younger children, tell them real food is good for us; it helps us stay healthy and not get sick. Use words like whole food or "growing food." This will help them differentiate between real food and refined, processed foods. As children get older, be more specific. They can start learning about different food categories, foods that are nutritious, and foods that aren't. They can learn about variety within each group. Share specific information about nutrients in foods and which foods are especially nutrient-dense. Talk about the dangers and health risks of eating unhealthful food. Help them make the connection between eating healthful food and feeling healthy, energetic, and nourished.

Balance: Try to maintain balance. It is important not to complicate your life so much that you give up. Think about the easiest areas to change and the most important (home, school lunches, snacks on the road, fast food for dinner, candy at the grocery store). Make changes and maintain them. But be careful of becoming too extreme. Forcing change can lead to resistance and defiance, and may backfire. Making people eat a certain way can cause them to crave the "forbidden food," and it may seem even more desirable.

Every family has to decide where to draw the line. At home, we have healthful, real foods. Sweet treats are saved for desserts or special occasions, but lollipops have saved the day many times. In other people's homes, we enjoy their company and their food. Kids can eat whatever they want, but I do try to limit soda and candy. We definitely lighten up when traveling and on vacation, but not too much. We learned the hard way that well-fed children are better-behaved children (and well-fed parents are better at parenting.) If we have to stop while we are out, we try to find a deli or restaurant instead of fast food.

Enjoyment: Real foods have a wonderful array of flavors, aromas, and textures. Find the best foods possible, learn how to cook them well, and enjoy satisfying, fulfilling meals. Sharing family meals together can be one of the best gifts you can give to your children. You nourish their bodies and their emotional health at the same time.

Tools for Avoiding Food Battles

The more I keep my mouth closed, the more my children open theirs. Author, dietitian, and therapist Ellyn Satter states, "The way to get a kid to eat is not to try. You have to let it be her idea. You shouldn't force your child to eat (or restrict the amount she eats.) It is the most unhelpful thing you can possibly do. To either of you." Along with following the division of responsibilities (parents provide food and children decide what and how much to eat), other tools and information may be helpful. If food battles become a significant issue, seek professional guidance.

Hunger Cycles: Become familiar with your children's hunger cycles and what they eat at each meal and snack. Use the information to help you manage the day. If lunch was early or small, have a substantial mid-afternoon snack such as soup, sandwich, or dinner leftovers. Some children are better eaters at different times of the day. If all meals and snacks are nutritious, this relieves the pressure of making one meal supply the bulk of nutrients. It may also be helpful to mix up the types of food served at meals. Have soup for breakfast or eggs for lunch.

> ** Experts disagree about the concept of "grazing" (eating frequent small meals and snacks throughout the day). Some feel it is the natural hunger cycle of the child and should be acknowledged. Others discourage grazing, stating it can interfere with a more nutritious meal. While it can be inconvenient to constantly feed hungry children healthful food throughout the day, I do my best to acknowledge hunger with nutritious food. Find ways to make life easier by saving unfinished snacks and leftovers meals for the next bout of hunger. Gently try to lengthen time in between meals and stretch hunger cycles with distracting, enjoyable activities. This becomes easier as children become older.*

Developmental Stages: Be aware of and flexible with the different developmental stages of children. At certain times children may become naturally suspicious of new foods. Or they may want the same food repeatedly. Then, there is every parent's favorite, the "I-don't-want-anything-to-touch" phase, where we diligently separate the peas, carrots, and corn into three separate piles from the bag of mixed vegetables.

I originally did not like the idea of "playing with food" (making designs and using cookie cutters) to encourage eating. Then I had picky eaters. If children will eat broccoli "trees," zucchini "grass," and sandwiches shaped like animals, do it. "Make Your Own Meals" (MYOM) like tacos, shish kebabs, and pizza that allow children to choose their own ingredients are usually popular too. Some health authorities recommend offering only one meal even if children refuse to eat it. They state that children should learn to eat the meal which has been prepared and not turn parents into short-order cooks. If I cook new foods, however, or something "unpopular," I am more flexible and try to have leftovers on hand. Everyone seems to appreciate another option when I am experimenting.

Repetition: Encourage children to try new foods. Allow them to take one bite and politely spit it into a napkin if they do not like it. Then ask them to take one bite and actually eat it. It may take 10 to 14 times of repeated exposure to a new food before a child will accept it. Keep offering and exposing children to new foods. Serve food family-style, passed around in bowls, where everyone helps themselves. Children can try just a "taste" or begin to judge amounts of food they think they will eat. When children routinely experience unfamiliar foods without pressure to eat them, they can be more open to experimenting.

Separate bowls of fun salad toppings is an excellent way to introduce new foods. Place salad greens on the table with small bowls of familiar favorites and new foods: cheeses, nuts, seeds, beans, grains, chopped fruit, dried fruit, or vegetables. Children may not like marinated beets at first but at least they will know what they look like, and hopefully, taste like. Exposure to new foods can be your initial goal. If they are eaten, it's a bonus.

Planning: Bring healthful snacks when going out and send children to school with nutritious lunches from home. Have rules about juice, snacks, sweet treats, or any food you might want to limit. Junk food is the same as other unsafe activities. I often hear that soda or candy "can't hurt." I believe it can and does, along with other fake and refined foods. It certainly doesn't help. Children will experiment as they get older. But surrounding them with healthful food at home and nutritious meals on the table lessens the impact and balances the negatives with positives.

Once we learn to appreciate the taste and nourishment of quality whole foods, so will our children. They are the ones, ultimately, who will decide what to eat as they get older. If we can help them trust their natural hunger cues and provide modeling, experience, knowledge, a sense of balance, and enjoyment, they will have a strong base of healthful habits to guide them. We need to make sure this generation of children grows up knowing about and eating real foods.

Safety and Equipment

Safety for Younger Children:
- never leave children unattended in the kitchen
- always wash hands prior to working with food
- dry hands for a good grip on cooking utensils
- be careful of long or loose clothing and apron strings
- tie back loose clothing and long hair
- have a first aid kit and fire extinguisher available
- unplug appliances when finished and keep them away from water
- turn pot and pan handles toward back of work area
- give children serrated or plastic knives to use only with adult supervision

Safety for Older Children:
- same as above
- hold knives and scissors by handles and cut away from the body
- place dirty knives in a safe place near the sink (soapy water can hide sharp blades)
- use potholders/oven mitts to handle hot pots and pans
- learn about proper food handling and storage

Equipment for Parents:
- blender: for smoothies and pureeing soups
- mixer: for breads and cookies
- food processor: for slicing, shredding, mincing, and grinding.
- cutting boards
- quality knives
- peeler, grater, brush, and garlic press
- oven mitt
- crockpot
- breadmaker
- juicer
- pressure cooker
- skillets and pots
- baking pans (cookie sheet, loaf, muffin, pie, cake, and roasting)
- bowls
- digital, instant read food thermometer

<u>Equipment for Children:</u>
- stable chair or stool
- measuring cups and spoons
- colander/strainer
- spoon, whisk, spatula, ladle, and rolling pin (child-size*)
- salad spinner
- aprons
- cookie cutters
- hard-boiled egg slicer (good for kiwi, strawberries, and other fruit instead of knives)
- melon baller
- toothpicks (colored for older kids)
- bowls (child-size*)
- baking pans (child-size: cookie sheet, loaf, muffin, pie, and cake*)
- timer

*See Equipment in Appendix C

Age Appropriate Activities (these are suggested activities—all children are developmentally different and parents should be the judge of a child's readiness)

Up to three years old:

Skills: building vocabulary, fine motor skills (mixing, mashing, etc.), eye-hand coordination, counting, sequencing, patience, confidence, and self esteem
- grocery shop/identify foods
- gather ingredients
- choose meals, snacks, ingredients, and/or flavors (type of fruit in a smoothie)
- measure, pour, mash, mix
- tear salad greens
- practice cutting clay with plastic knives
- push appliance buttons
- "set" table
- "wash" and/or dry appropriate dishes
- "load" dishwasher

- set timer
- taste test

Younger Children:

Skills: reading, math (measuring, fractions, etc.), fine motor skills, further language development (describing, predicting, following directions, sequencing, etc.), science (cause and effect, temperature, etc.), patience, confidence, creativity, and self esteem

- parent as helper, when possible (see *Pretend Soup* in *Recommended Reading* section)
- help plan menu
- grocery shop
- gather ingredients
- choose meals, snacks, ingredients, and/or flavors
- measure, pour, mash, mix
- use appliances (with supervision)
- cut soft foods with serrated knife (with supervision)
- crack eggs into separate bowl/check for shells
- choose, read, and follow recipes
- learn stove and oven basics
- learn about storing foods properly
- learn about "doneness" of foods (judging when food is finished cooking)
- set and clear the table
- help with dishes/clean up

Older Children:

Skills: further reading, math, language, and science skills, self esteem, confidence, creativity, and independence

- plan menu
- shop
- choose, read, and follow recipes
- practice stove and oven basics (with supervision that isn't obvious)
- use appliances
- cut, chop
- learn to test when food is done

- learn to keep produce and raw meats separate
- wash hands, utensils, and cutting boards after handling raw meats
- learn about storing foods properly
- set and clear the table
- help with dishes/clean up

Afterword

As my knowledge and experience with real food continues to grow, so does my respect, appreciation, and awe. The importance and power of consuming nutrient-dense foods is nothing short of miraculous. Our society has become disconnected, disrespectful, and neglectful of our natural food resources. But there are hopeful signs: the spread of sustainable community farms, the increase in animals returned to pasture, and the rapid growth of the health food market.

As with any growing industry, there are many people anxious to become involved. Some are motivated by the desire to produce high-quality nutrient-dense foods the best way possible. They have a respect for nature and the potential of real foods. Others will be tempted to compromise and cut corners. It is our job to know the difference.

This book focuses on understanding healthful foods and shifting to a more healthful way of eating. I have tried to remain consistent with this message and not diverge into discussions of corporate bullying, manipulative advertising to children, and other ethical or political topics. But these are important issues. They are delicately and critically interwoven into the fabric of healthful eating and need to be addressed: soda companies offering financially desperate school systems large amounts of money in return for making vending machines accessible to children; the marriage of celebrities, athletes, and cartoon characters to unhealthful food products, and industry's behind-the-scenes wheeling and dealing with government. Some parents may choose to focus their efforts, energy, and money on supporting the producers of high-quality real foods, hoping those who do not will naturally die out. Others may choose to take a more active role. (See *Recommend Reading* for suggestions.)

As parents we are responsible for protecting our children. Unhealthful food harms children. What kind of society will we be if continually produce increasingly unhealthy generations? We need to reverse the "P" generation cycle and reconnect children to real foods. We can change this destructive course and move towards a healthier society.

> *"If we don't change direction,*
> *we will end up precisely where we are heading."*
> —Old Chinese Proverb

Refined to Real Food
Fixing Real Foods:
Quick Ideas and Basic Recipes

BREAKFASTS

Quick Ideas	Recipes
Sprouted Grain Toast with Toppings	Easy Omelet
Eggs with Leftover Vegetables	Fast Frittata
Soup, Sandwich, or Leftover Dinner	Hearty Hot Cereal
Whole Grain "Traditional" Breakfasts	Strawberry Banana Smoothie
Better Bacon & Sausage	Peach Yogurt Smoothie

LUNCHES, SALADS, AND SOUPS

Quick Ideas	Recipes
Nut Butter & Jelly (NBJ)	Chicken Salad
Three-bean Salad	Grain & Bean Salad
Pasta Vegetable Salad	Salad Greens with Toppings
Better Lunch Meat & Hot Dogs	Lentil & Rice Soup
Lunchbox Ideas	Black Bean & Corn Soup

DINNERS

Quick Ideas	Recipes
Broiled White Fish Fillets	Snappy Salmon
Pastas	Mainstream Meatloaf
Chili	Hearty Slow Cooker Stew
Rubs, Roasts & Grilling	Simple Stir-Fry
Make Your Own Meals	Basic Burrito

VEGETABLES, SIDES, AND SAUCES

Quick Ideas	Recipes
Steamed Fresh Vegetables	Roasted Vegetables
Sautéed Greens	Ratatouille
Marinated Grilled Vegetables	Pilaf Pizzazz
Pineapple Sweet Potatoes	Baked Stuffed Squash
Grain and Bean Side Dishes	Tahini Dressing

SNACKS AND DESSERTS

Quick Ideas	Recipes
Trail Mix	Maple Zucchini Bread
Whole Grain Breads & Toppings	Banana Molasses Bread
Produce & Dips	Apple Crisp
Nachos with Salsa, Beans, and Cheese	Carrot Cake
Frozen Treats	Apple Fig Bars

Fixing Real Foods:
Quick Ideas and Basic Recipes

Cooking can be challenging enough, but work, children, and outside responsibilities can make it seem impossible. At a time when it is most critical for young children to eat properly, it is also when we have the least amount of time. Use your children's health as a source of motivation and inspiration to find ways to prepare nutritious foods.

These recipes are a sampling of the wide range of possibilities for using real foods. The trick with cooking is to learn a few basic techniques that can be easily adapted to create new and interesting dishes. "Quick Ideas" are gentle reminders about simple foods that can be made without much instruction. "Basic Recipes" provide detailed information as well as variations and tips.

Start with foods, snacks, and meals you and your family already enjoy and make them more healthful. Then write down foods you would like to try next. If weeknights are too hectic, set aside time to prepare meals during the weekend. It can actually be more efficient to plan ahead, shop, and cook all at one time. Place fish, chicken, or other meats with marinades in sealed bags in the freezer. Remove and defrost in the refrigerator the day before. Make big batches of chili, soup, stew, and meatloaf so that you have leftovers on hand.

For those new to the kitchen or looking to improve their skills, quality cookbooks can be beneficial. Also try subscriptions to cooking magazines, tape cooking shows on television, take cooking classes, ask friends and family members for favorite recipes, and look in the local library for cookbooks and instructional videos. As your knowledge of cooking real foods continues to grow, so can your recipe box* and cookbook library (see Appendix D).

Don't force yourself or your family to eat foods you don't like. Find real foods you do like and prepare them in great-tasting ways so that you love to eat them. You should feel nourished and satisfied after a meal.

A three-ring binder with clear plastic insert pages can be a useful tool. Copy and insert favorite recipes, removing old or unused copies as needed. When cooking from a recipe, remove the page from the binder and tape to a cabinet at eye level. It will not use up valuable counter space or be affected by spills.

Breakfasts: Quick Ideas

This meal sets the stage for the rest of your day. Make it balanced and healthful. Look for ways to include quality sources of proteins, fats, and carbohydrates, and maybe even those elusive vegetables.

<u>Sprouted Grain Toast with Toppings:</u> There are various sprouted grain breads and bread products available. Try Ezekiel bread or other varieties (see "Favorite Foods List" p.164). Top with nut butter, cottage cheese, or a poached egg.

<u>Scrambled Eggs with Leftover Vegetables:</u> Cook extra vegetables at dinner and mix leftovers with eggs in the morning. Wrap in a tortilla, put in a pita, or just eat as is! This is also a great way to use up lingering produce in the vegetable bin.

<u>Soup, Sandwich, or Leftover Dinner:</u> Soup, sandwiches, or leftovers from a favorite meal are great ways to start the day. Look for slow-cooker soup recipes that can cook while you sleep—a nice treat in winter. Switch to smoothies in the summer.

<u>Whole Grain "Traditional" Breakfasts:</u> Switch your traditional refined grain breakfast to whole-grain and high-fiber versions. Top cereal with berries (lower on the glycemic index than other fruits), nuts, or ground flax seeds. Make sure your pancake mix, waffles, bagels, and other bread products are whole grain too. Top with yogurt or nut butters for added protein and nutrients.

<u>"Better" Bacon and Sausage:</u> Find products free of hormones, antibiotics, nitrates, and other meat preservatives. Many quality products are now being made from turkey and chicken too. They can add a great source of protein to a traditionally all-carbohydrate breakfast (see "Favorite Foods List" p. 164).
See also "Breads" in "Snacks & Desserts."

Easy Omelet

A basic breakfast recipe everyone should know. Also a quick, easy lunch or dinner for a change.—AA

1 teaspoon butter
2 eggs
1 tablespoon milk, cream, or water (optional)
Salt and freshly ground black pepper to taste
2/3 cup leftover, cooked vegetables
1/4 cup shredded Cheddar cheese (about 1 ounce)

Melt the butter in a small skillet on medium-high heat to coat. (Sauté vegetables to heat through if desired.) Beat the eggs, milk, salt, and pepper in a small bowl. Pour the mixture into the skillet and cook until it begins to set, about 30 to 60 seconds. Tip the skillet slightly, moving the cooked egg to center while allowing the uncooked, runny egg mixture to run along the sides of the skillet. When the egg has set, add the vegetables and cheese on top. Fold in half and slide onto a plate.

Serves 1

Variations:

- Add 1 tablespoon fresh or 1 teaspoon dried herbs: parsley, oregano, or basil.
- Add other vegetables: diced tomatoes or strips of dark leafy greens.
- Try diced meats: ham, bacon, or sausage.
- Add a natural salsa at the end for extra flavor.

Tip: A nonstick skillet makes cooking omelets even easier.

Tip: If you have no leftover vegetables, sauté fresh just before cooking: onions, mushrooms, and peppers work well.

Tip: This is a great way to use up extra vegetables left in the refrigerator bin.

Fast Frittata

My husband will often make this frittata as a Sunday morning
treat. He uses whatever vegetables we have on hand. For the two of
us, this can be quite large, but leftovers are wonderful too. —ST

1 tablespoon butter
1 cup cooked, chopped vegetables (peppers, mushrooms, onions)
6 to 8 eggs
1/4 cup heavy cream
3/4 teaspoon freshly ground black pepper
1 teaspoon seasoning mix
1/2 cup shredded extra sharp Cheddar cheese (about 2 ounces)
1/2 cup shredded fontina cheese (about 2 ounces)

Melt the butter in large skillet on low-medium heat. Add the vegetables and sauté lightly to warm. In a medium bowl, whisk the eggs, cream, pepper, and seasoning until well mixed. Pour the egg mixture over the evenly distributed vegetables. Cook over low-medium heat for 10 to 15 minutes until the edges begin to firm. Do not stir. Evenly distribute the cheeses on top of the cooking egg mixture. Cover and let cook for another 10 to 15 minutes until the cheeses melt and the eggs become firm.

Serves 4

Variations:

- Vary your vegetables: try asparagus, broccoli, shredded greens, or zucchini.
- Add egg whites instead of whole eggs.
- Use milk, soymilk, or half-and-half instead of heavy cream.
- Use another high-moisture, white cheese instead of fontina (like Gruyère or Gouda).
- Or bake in the oven at 350° for 25 to 30 minutes, uncovered

Tip: Sprinkle a dash of paprika over the cooked frittata for added color and flavor.

Tip: Also look for quiche recipes. These make great lunches and dinners too!

Hearty Hot Cereal

So warming, filling, and nutritious compared to cold cereals. How nice to wake to a warm breakfast, and the additions are endless!
—AA

1 cup rolled oats
1/3 cup raisins
1/2 teaspoon cinnamon, or other sweetener
2 cups water
pinch of salt

Bring water to a boil in a medium saucepan. Add the oats, raisins, salt, and cinnamon. Cover, reduce heat to low, and simmer until water is absorbed, about 10 minutes.

Serves 2

Variations:

- Add other chopped, dried fruits: apricots, dates, figs, or prunes.
- Try chopped nuts: almonds, pecans, or walnuts.
- Add fresh fruits after cooking: apples, berries, or peaches.
- Try other sweeteners: vanilla, cream, maple syrup, or honey.
- Try less-processed oats such as steel-cut, Irish, or Scotch oats (use 3 cups of water and triple the cooking time or soak over night).
- Experiment with other whole-grain, hot cereals: rolled or flaked grains or mixed, cracked grains.

Tip: Cook grains overnight in a slow cooker and wake up to a warm meal already prepared.

Tip: Cook grains in the morning while exercising or showering, puree in a processor with milk or cream and sweet spices. Top with fresh fruit.

Tip: Other warming spices include nutmeg, cloves, and allspice. Use smaller amounts of nutmeg and cloves as they are quite potent.

Strawberry Banana Smoothie

*Smoothies are a blended fruit drink typically made with fruit and
milk or yogurt. I prefer using a frozen banana for a dairy-free
version with the same cool, creamy consistency.—AA*

1 cup water or juice
1 1/2 cups strawberries, frozen
1 small banana, frozen, sliced into chunks
1 teaspoon cashew butter

Pour the liquid into a blender.
Add the fruit and cashew butter.
Blend until smooth, about 30 seconds.
Serves 2

Variations:

- Substitute other fruits: cherries, peaches, or pineapple for the
  strawberries, or try a combination of fruits.
- Try different liquids: juices, milks, or yogurt. They can add other
  nutrients as well as a different taste. (Juice is popular, but adds
  extra sugar and contains less fiber.)
- Try other nut and seed butters: almond, peanut, or tahini (cashew
  tends to be thicker and easier to use).

Tip: Leave your blender out on the counter. Digging in the back of
a cabinet for an awkward appliance can easily derail plans for a
healthful snack.

Tip: Use small amounts of frozen blueberries or ice cubes to
thicken drinks.

Tip: Buy extra fruit, especially ripe fruit on sale. Peel, slice, and
freeze it so you always have some on hand.

Peach Yogurt Smoothie
I have this several times a week for breakfast. Add one scoop of protein powder and a teaspoon of flax oil, and I'm set for the morning! —AA

1 cup orange juice
2/3 cup vanilla yogurt
1 ½ cup peaches, frozen
½ -1 cups raspberries, frozen (or blueberries)

Place the juice, yogurt, and fruit in a blender.
Blend until smooth, about 30 seconds.
Serves 2

Variations:
- Try other fruits: apricots, mangoes, and blueberries work well. (Drained, canned fruit may also be used. Ice cubes or sherbet help thicken, bind, and cool the smoothie.)
- Try other juices, milks, or other flavorful yogurts.
- For additional flavor, add 1/2 teaspoon of vanilla, cinnamon, or honey.
- For added protein, try small amounts of soft cubed tofu, nut butter, or protein powder.

Tip: A "dishwasher safe" blender can save time and energy. Or try filling the container halfway with warm water and a drop of dish soap. Blend for 30 seconds. Rinse.

Tip: Buy cases of frozen, organic fruit when they go on sale.

Tip: Smoothies are a great way to add supplements (ground flax seeds, flax oil, calcium, protein powders, or "green food"). Too many supplements, however, can make smoothies undrinkable.

Lunches, Soups, and Salads: Quick Ideas

Many people eat lunch "on the go." Whether for work or school, these recipes emphasize foods that can travel. Find travel-worthy equipment and containers: ice packs to keep foods cold, thermoses to keep foods hot, and small plastic containers for dips and make-your-own (MYO)-type lunches (see "Equipment" in Appendix C).

Nut Butter and Jelly (NBJ): Make this kid favorite even more nutritious. Use whole grain or sprouted grain bread, natural or organic nut butters (almond and cashew are popular), and an all-natural jelly or jam.

Three-bean Salad: Drain one or more cans of beans (black, pinto, and white, or green, yellow wax, and kidney), add chopped green or red pepper, onion, and garlic, a can of corn (if desired), fresh herbs (parsley or cilantro), salt and freshly ground black pepper to taste, and toss with your favorite olive oil and vinegar dressing.

Pasta Vegetable Salad: An easy favorite and a great way to sneak in extra vegetables. Toss favorite pasta (whole grain if possible) with cherry tomatoes, chopped peppers, red onions, olive oil, vinegar, and basil or parsley. Also try zucchini, olives, and other vegetables and herbs for variety.

Better Lunch Meat and Hot Dogs: Look for better-quality lunch meats and hot dogs without antibiotics, hormones, or nitrates. Products made from chicken, turkey, and even salmon as well as beef are also available.

Lunchbox Ideas: Dried fruit, nuts, whole-grain cereal, fresh fruit, minifoods (muffins, meatloaves, and quiches), wraps, pita pockets, cheeses, leftovers (stir-fry, chili, and stew); see also "Snacks and Desserts."

Chicken Salad

We often enjoy roasted chicken and always make extra for salad.
There are numerous variations of this recipe. This one is our
favorite.—ST

2 to 3 cups cooked chicken, chopped (roasted, skinless is best)
1/2 cup chopped dried cranberries
1/2 cup chopped roasted walnuts
1 cup cucumber, peeled, de-seeded, and chopped
2 to 3 tablespoons mayonnaise
1 to 2 teaspoons Dijon mustard
Salt and freshly ground black pepper to taste

Mix all of the ingredients in a medium bowl.
Transfer to a covered container and keep refrigerated.
Serves 4-6

Variations:
• Try on sprouted grain bread, in pita pockets, or in wraps.
• Substitute other dried fruits and nuts.
•Try light mayonnaise
• Use turkey instead of chicken.

Tip: Keep some type of salad on hand: tuna, egg, or "Mock Egg Salad" made with tofu.

Tip: Use on top of salad greens or add dark leafy greens to the pocket, wrap, or sandwich.

Tip: Make extra chicken and turkey at dinner. Use leftovers for salads.

Grain and Bean Salad

This is a great way to use whole grains, beans, and vegetables.
Start with rice, canned beans, and a bottled vinaigrette. Add
vegetables, and it's done. Move on to other grains, cooked beans,
and homemade dressings when you are ready.—AA

2 cups brown rice, cooked (or other grain)
1 cup black beans, cooked (or one 15-ounce can, drained)
1 green pepper, chopped
1 tomato, chopped
1/2 cup red onion chopped
1/2 cup vinaigrette dressing
2 tablespoons chopped fresh parsley
Salt and freshly ground black pepper to taste

Toss all ingredients together in a bowl. Refrigerate and serve.
Serves 4 to 6

Variations:

• Try other grains: barley, quinoa, and wild rice.
• Use other beans: kidney, chickpeas, and pinto beans.
• Use other fruits and vegetables: avocado, olives, raisins, grapes, or
   citrus fruits.
• Experiment with other herbs and spices: basil, cilantro, or mint.
• Experiment with other dressings.

Tip: Have extra grains and beans on hand for use in soups, salads,
   and pilafs. (For a pilaf, sauté vegetables and add cooked grains
   and beans until heated through.)

Tip: Cook grains in stock for added flavor.

Tip: Cook extra grains in the morning, at dinner, or on the
   weekend and refrigerate. Use half for a salad and half for a pilaf.

Salad Greens with Toppings

We have salad every night with dinner. It is quick and automatic now—slice a few strips off romaine hearts, add some spinach or other bagged, mixed greens, and put toppings into bowls, salad-bar style.
—AA.

Salad Greens

<u>Toppings</u>

Fruits: Apples, pears, tangerines, olives, and raspberries

Vegetables: Cucumbers, peppers, onions, tomatoes, and mushrooms

Beans: Chickpeas, black beans, pinto beans, and other beans

Cheeses: Feta, cheddar, parmesan, and other cheeses (grated, crumbled, or shredded)

Nuts: Chopped almonds, cashews, pecans, and other nuts

Seeds: Pine nuts, pumpkin, sunflower, sesame, and other seeds

Wash and dry greens. Tear or slice. Add toppings and dressing.

Variations:

- Try other greens: arugula, bibb lettuce, butterhead lettuce, cabbages, chard, greens (beet, dandelion, or mustard), leaf lettuces, mixed greens, or watercress.
- Find special pairings you enjoy: pears and raspberries, tangerines and black olives, or apples and walnuts.
- A great way to get seeds into your diet: put in a bowl and sprinkle on salad or other dinner foods.

Tip: Prewashed, bagged greens can save time and energy on busy nights.

Tip: Washing and tearing greens is a great kid's job. Or roll and slice larger greens into strips if on your own or short on time.

Tip: Spinach tends to be sandy, so wash it well. Salad spinners are great for helping to dry wet, washed greens, or use a colander.

Lentil & Rice Soup

I can put this soup together now in about ten minutes (if my kids aren't "helping"). They like it thick, so it will stick to their spoons and is easy to eat. For a "thinner" soup, add less rice or more broth. —AA

1 tablespoon olive oil

1 onion, minced

1 garlic clove, minced

8 cups chicken broth or vegetable broth

1 cup red lentils, washed

1 cup brown rice

4 medium carrots, sliced

4 celery stalks, sliced

1 teaspoon seasoning mix

1 teaspoon dried parsley

Add the oil to a large soup pot over medium heat. Sauté the onions for 1 minute. Add the garlic and heat for 1 minute more. Pour in the broth, lentils, rice, carrots, celery, and seasonings. Bring to a boil then simmer, covered, for 1 hour until vegetables are tender.

Serves 6 to 8

Variations:

- Use different types of lentils or split peas. (For split pea soup: sauté vegetables, add 2 cups of split peas, 8 cups of broth, and seasonings. Bring to a boil, simmer 2 hours. Puree half or all of the soup for a thick, creamy texture.)
- Try other grains like quinoa, buckwheat, or none at all.
- Vary your vegetables: try adding quick-cooking greens such as spinach at the end.

Tip: Buy organic chicken broth (32-fluid-ounce aseptic boxes) in bulk when it goes on sale.

Tip: Store in a sealed container for 3 to 4 days in the refrigerator or freeze half for later.

Tip: Order stainless vacuum snack jars from Gold Mine Natural Foods (see "Equipment" in Appendix C). Their wide mouths and compact size (9.5 ounces) are perfect for soups, whether traveling or in lunch boxes.

Black Bean and Corn Soup

Learning how to make basic soups is time well invested. It is another great way to include whole grains, vegetables, and beans, formerly the hardest foods to get into my diet.—AA

1 tablespoon olive oil
2 medium onions, chopped
3 to 4 garlic cloves, minced
3 cups black beans, cooked
8 cups chicken stock (or vegetable)
1 (15-ounce) can corn, drained
2 teaspoons lemon or lime juice
1/2 teaspoon dried oregano
Salt and freshly ground black pepper to taste

Add the oil to a large soup pot over medium heat. Sauté the onions for 2 to 3 minutes until tender. Add the garlic and heat for 1 minute more. Pour in the beans, stock, corn, lemon juice, oregano, salt, and pepper. Bring to a boil then simmer for 15-20 minutes. Puree half of the soup for a creamy texture (see Tip).

Serves 6 to 8

Variations:

- Add other vegetables: carrots, celery, or strips of dark leafy greens.
- Try other spices or herbs: cumin, parsley, or crushed red pepper flakes.
- For additional flavor, use diced bacon instead of oil and sauté the onion in the drippings.

Tip: Look for other soup recipes: chicken, minestrone, mushroom and barley, or other favorites.

Tip: Get the soup started when you first wake up and let it simmer while you shower. It's a warm way to start the day or have soup ready for later.

Tip: Be careful when pureeing soups. If the blender is too full, hot liquids can explode. (Some food processors leak through the middle, and immersion blenders spray if you lift them too far out of the pot.)

Dinners: Quick Ideas

The focus of these meals is on basic recipes that, once mastered, require little thought after a long, tiring day. Add steamed vegetables and a salad and you're done. There are also suggestions for make your own meals (MYOM). Individuals choose their own ingredients and assemble their own dishes. (If kids create them, they are more likely to eat them.)

<u>Baked White Fish Fillets:</u> Coat with melted butter and bread crumbs. Bake at 375° for 15 – 20 minutes until it flakes with a fork. Sprinkle with fresh lemon juice, add a salsa or sauce, and place on bed of sautéed greens.

<u>Pastas:</u> Spaghetti, lasagna, tortellini, stuffed shells—the possibilities are endless, and pasta is usually a favorite with children. Use it as an opportunity to improve nutrition. Try whole-grain pastas, added vegetables and/or quality meats, with a flavorful sauce.

<u>Chili:</u> A quick chili can be cooked with ground beef, beans, tomato sauce, and a little chili powder. For more variety, try other ground meats (turkey, chicken, or pork), shredded chicken, beans, chopped onions, garlic, peppers, other vegetables, and spices such as oregano and cumin. Top with grated cheese and serve with corn bread.

<u>Rubs, Roasts, and Grilling:</u> "Rub" meat, poultry, or seafood with your favorite spices and flavorings. Roast in the oven, cook on the grill, or place in slow cooker—a quick and easy way to prepare many entrées. (See "Herbs and Spices" in Appendix B.)

<u>Make Your Own Meals (MYOM):</u> Children love choices. Leave out nutritious fixings (cooked meats, beans, chopped fruits and vegetables, cheeses, salsas, and bread choices) and let them assemble their own meals. Try burritos, fajitas, pizzas, quesadillas, shish kebabs, and tacos. They are more likely to eat their own creations.

Snappy Salmon
This classic marinade can be used with meat, fish, and poultry.
—AA

Marinade:

1/4 cup olive oil

3 tablespoons soy sauce

2 cloves garlic, minced

1 teaspoon honey

2 tablespoons lemon or orange juice

Freshly ground black pepper to taste

4 salmon fillets (4 to 6 ounces each)

In a medium bowl, whisk together the marinade ingredients. Marinate the fillets for 1 hour in the refrigerator, in a shallow baking dish or zipper-type bag. Broil the fillets, skin side down, until the edges flake and the center is still slightly red (5 to 10 minutes depending on thickness—fish will continue cooking after it is removed from heat).

Serves 4

Variations:

• Use other sweeteners in place of honey: sugar or maple syrup.

• Replace lemon juice: vinegars and white wine are popular.

• Try sesame oil in place of olive oil.

Tip: Enjoy fresh, wild salmon throughout the summer (king, sockeye, or coho.) Choose from frozen or farmed during the off-season.

Tip: Fillets are usually thinner and cook faster. The skin can be easily removed after cooking. Some small "pin bones" may also need to be removed. Steaks are thicker, can be easily grilled, and need to be turned.

Tip: Also try baking, poaching, and other fish recipes.

Mainstream Meatloaf

Another classic meal. Learn a basic recipe, experiment with variations, and make extras to freeze.—AA

1 1/2 - 2 pounds lean ground meat (beef or turkey)
2 egg
1 cup onion, chopped
1 cup celery, chopped (about 2 to 3 large ribs)
2 garlic cloves, minced
1 cup bread crumbs
1/2 cup grated Parmesan cheese (about 2 ounces)
1 cup milk
3 tablespoons chopped fresh parsley, or 1 tablespoon dried
Salt and freshly ground black pepper to taste

Preheat oven to 350° and grease a 9 x 5-inch loaf pan with butter, oil, or spray. Combine all the ingredients in large bowl and mix with hands until blended. Mold into the loaf pan and place on the center rack in the oven. Bake for 1 to 1 1/4 hours, or until center temperature reaches 160°. Let stand for 5 to 10 minutes before slicing.

Serves 4 to 6

Variations:

- Add other chopped vegetables: carrots, peppers, squash, or zucchini.
- Try other fresh or dried herbs, seasonings, and flavorings: thyme, sage, Worcestershire sauce, or mustard.
- Try rolled oats in place of bread crumbs.
- Try ketchup in place of milk.

Tip: Grease muffin tins for miniloaves and faster cooking.

Tip: Cooked meatloaves freeze well. Double or triple the recipe.

Tip: Leftovers make great sandwiches.

Hearty Slow-Cooker Stew

There is nothing better than coming home after a long day to the smell of a wonderful dinner already made.—ST

1 pound cubed beef
1 cup cubed turnip
2 medium red potatoes, cubed
1 medium onion, chopped
2 garlic cloves, minced
3 large carrots, sliced
2 bay leaves
2 teaspoons dried thyme
3 tablespoons tomato paste
1/2 teaspoon celery salt
1/2 teaspoon freshly ground black pepper
1 quart organic beef broth or bouillon

Place the meat, vegetables, seasonings, and broth in a slow cooker. Cover and cook on low for 6 to 8 hours. Remove the bay leaves and serve.

Serves 4 to 6

Variations:

• Use cubed stew beef or other meats.
• Try other vegetables: add sliced greens or frozen peas 30 minutes before serving.
• Try different broths: chicken, vegetable, or mushroom.
Tip: Chop the ingredients the night before and refrigerate. Place in a slow cooker the next morning (don't forget to turn it on!) and come home to hot dinner ready to serve.
Tip: Browning the cubed beef first helps to seal in flavors.
Tip: If you have a bread maker with a timer, stew and bread can be ready at the same time.

Basic Stir-Fry

This recipe has endless variations. Make sure all the ingredients are ready next to the cooktop. Once you get cooking, it goes fast!—AA

<u>Sauce</u>
1 tablespoon cornstarch
1/2 cup chicken broth (or water)
1 teaspoon honey (or sugar)
1 tablespoon soy sauce
2 tablespoons peanut oil (or sesame)
2 garlic cloves, minced
1 teaspoon minced ginger (optional)
<u>Stir-Fry</u>
2 tablespoon coconut oil (or other high heat oil)
1 pound chicken, thinly sliced
3 cups thinly sliced vegetables (carrots, celery, peppers)

Combine cornstarch and broth. Blend well. Mix in other ingredients for the sauce in a medium bowl until dissolved. Set aside. Place a large, heavy skillet over high heat and add 1 tablespoons of coconut oil. Stir-fry the meat 3 to 4 minutes, or until tender. Remove from the skillet. Add the remaining oil and longest-cooking vegetables (carrots and celery), and stir-fry for 1 minute. Continue adding vegetables and cook until crisp and tender. Return the chicken to the skillet. Add the cornstarch mixture. Stir until thick and coated.

Serves 4 to 6

Variations:

- Meat: try shrimp, beef, or tofu (marinate tofu for 1 hour).
- Vegetables: try asparagus, broccoli, cabbage, cauliflower, greens, snow peas, squash, water chestnuts, or zucchini.
- Sauce: add 1 teaspoon sesame oil, vinegar (balsamic, cider, or rice wine), or try different broths and reduced-sodium soy sauce

Tip: Serve over brown rice or noodles. Top with cashews.

Tip: Arrange sliced vegetables in order of time needed to cook; the longest time should be first.

Tip: A food processor helps slice uniform pieces that cook evenly and saves time.

Basic Burrito
A great Make-Your-Own-Meal kids love.—AA

4 flour tortillas
2 to 3 cups refried beans (two 15-ounce cans)
2 cups chopped lettuce
1 cup chopped tomato (about 2 medium tomatoes)
1 cup black olives, sliced
1 large onion, chopped
1 cup salsa
1 cup shredded Cheddar cheese (1/4 pound)
1/2 cup sour cream

Preheat the oven to 300°. Wrap the tortillas in foil and warm in the oven for 10 to 15 minutes. (Or place between two damp cloths and microwave for 30 to 60 seconds.) Heat the refried beans in a saucepan. Place the chopped vegetables in individual bowls. Put all the ingredients out buffet-style and let everyone build burritos with tortillas, beans, condiments, and cheese.

Serves 4

Variations:
- Try whole-grain or sprouted-grain tortillas. Replace flour tortillas with corn tortillas and make tacos (cooked, ground meat may be used in place of beans).
- Add other vegetables: peppers, mushrooms, shredded zucchini, or other types of lettuce and greens.
- Use other beans: kidney or pinto.
- Try other cheeses.
- Try other fillings: shredded chicken or pork, tofu, or rice.

Tip: Use canned refried beans or make ahead of time with a little cumin or chili powder.

Tip: Also try enchiladas or other baked wraps. Roll the ingredients (cooked meats, poultry, beans, vegetables, cheeses, salsas and other flavorings) in flour tortillas and place in a baking dish.

Cover with cheese, bake at 350° until cheese is melted (about 15 minutes), and serve.

Tip: Fajitas are another popular MYOM-type dish made with marinated meat, chicken, or fish, grilled vegetables, and an assortment of sides such as lettuce, tomatoes, sour cream, guacamole, or salsa, to build for yourself on flour tortillas.

Vegetables, Sides, and Sauces: Quick Ideas

This section offers ideas to help round out your meals and include a wider variety of whole grains and vegetables. Fresh steamed vegetables or cooked whole grains can be a treat by themselves or with a sauce. Find foods and recipes you love and make meal times more enjoyable.

Steamed Fresh Vegetables: Enjoy the flavor of fresh, quality produce. If looking for a little extra flavor, try grated Parmesan or other cheeses, a dash of butter or olive oil, or a sprinkling of sesame seeds. Each season has its own specialties.

Sautéed Greens (Bed of Greens): Perfect as a side dish or under fish, chicken, or other prepared entrée. Heat a skillet, add olive oil, onion, garlic, and greens (chard and spinach work well). Sauté for 1 to 2 minutes. Add a dash of soy sauce, maybe some nuts or seeds, or other seasoning. A great way to get those dark leafy greens!

Marinated Grilled Vegetables: When marinating meats or fish, get into the habit of reserving some marinade for grilled vegetables, too. Make a separate bowl or pouch for large slices of zucchini, eggplant, carrots, peppers, portobella mushrooms or more. You're already at the grill, be efficient and have a tasty side dish!

Pineapple Sweet Potatoes: Bake or boil sweet potatoes or yams until tender. Scoop out the flesh and mash with butter, crushed pineapple, and a dash of cinnamon. Add extra pineapple juice to thin, if desired. Leftover pineapple can be used in breads or muffins.

Grain or Bean Side Dishes: Cook up extra grains at breakfast. Use them as a side dish or a base under an entrée at dinner. Try barley, quinoa, or different types of rice. Add a flavorful sauce if enticements are desired. Use canned, baked beans or refried beans to start, then develop your own special recipes. Try other beans as a side dish, mixed into a pilaf, or on a salad.

Roasted Vegetables

A great way to include (or use up) a lot of vegetables. The trick is timing the slow-cooking and quick-cooking vegetables. Slice "slow cookers" small and "quick cookers" big (or add them at the end).—AA

Slow-Cooking Vegetables
  8 new potatoes, diced
  4 carrots, diced
  1 onion, diced
Quick-Cooking Vegetables
  2 green peppers, chunked
  2 yellow squash, chunked
  2 zucchini, chunked
Dressing:
  1/4 cup olive oil
  3 tablespoons lemon juice
  3 garlic cloves, minced
  1 teaspoon of oregano
  Salt and freshly ground black pepper to taste

Preheat the oven to 450°. Combine the vegetables in a large baking dish. In small bowl, whisk together the olive oil, lemon juice, garlic, oregano, salt, and pepper. Drizzle over the vegetables and toss to coat. Roast uncovered for 20 to 30 minutes, stirring once.

Serves 4 to 6

Variations:

- Use other fresh or dried herbs: basil, parsley, rosemary, or thyme.
- Use other vegetables: celery, mushrooms, snow peas, parsnips, or sweet potatoes.

Tip: Leftovers taste great.

Tip: Add slow-cooking vegetables to the pan when roasting poultry or meat.

Tip: For a quick side dish, use all quick-cooking vegetables, slice small, and cut cooking time in half.

Ratatouille

This is an end-of-the-summer ritual passed down from my father. It is a great way to manage all the late-summer tomatoes and zucchinis (and how it all started). We serve it with grated cheese on top.—AA

4 strips bacon, cut into pieces
1 onion, diced
1 green pepper, diced
1 red pepper, diced
3 garlic cloves, minced
3 cups diced tomatoes (about 2 pounds)
3 cups diced yellow squash (about 1 pound)
3 cups diced zucchini (about 1 pound)
2 teaspoons dried dill
Salt and freshly ground black pepper to taste
Parmesan cheese, grated (optional)

In large stew pot, fry the bacon until crisp. Add the onion, peppers, and garlic. Sauté for 2 to 3 minutes Add the tomatoes, squash, zucchini, dill, salt, and pepper. Simmer 15 to 20 minutes, or until all vegetables are tender. Top each serving with cheese.

Serves 8 to 10

Variations:

- Olive oil may be used instead of bacon.
- Add other vegetables: eggplant, mushrooms, or corn sliced off the cob.
- Use different herbs: fresh or dried basil, oregano, or parsley.
- Top with other cheeses: grated Cheddar, Swiss, or Romano.

Tip: This dish can also be cooked in the oven, but omit eggplant or sauté first in olive oil, onion, and garlic for 10 minutes. Bake at 350° for 45 minutes.

Tip: This recipe requires a lot of chopping but also yields a lot of food which freezes well.

Pilaf Pizzazz

Jazz up rice or other grain side dishes with some sautéed vegetables and beans. Use rice and canned beans to start, then branch out for greater variety and nutrients.—AA

1 tablespoon butter or oil
1 medium onion, chopped
1 red or green pepper, chopped
1 cup black beans, rinsed
1 cup corn
2 cups cooked brown rice
2 tablespoons soy sauce
Freshly ground black pepper to taste

Heat a large skillet over medium heat and melt the butter in it. Sauté the onion and pepper about 1 to 2 minutes. Add the beans, corn, rice, soy sauce, and pepper. Stir until heated through.

Serves 4 to 6

Variations:

- Use other chopped vegetables: mushrooms, water chestnuts, thawed frozen peas, celery, or tomatoes.
- Use other grains: barley, quinoa, buckwheat, or wild rice (cook in stock for added flavor).
- Use other beans: kidney, pinto, or navy.
- Use herbs to season: parsley, oregano, or thyme.
- Sprinkle with raisins, pine nuts, or other chopped dried fruits, nuts, and seeds.

Tip: When cooking rice or other grains, make extra for pilafs and salads (see tip below).

Tip: Use similar ingredients (grains, vegetables, and beans) with 1/4 cup of your favorite vinaigrette and fresh herb (parsley, basil, or cilantro) for a great-tasting salad.

Tip: Also look for recipes for fried rice, Spanish rice, and risotto.

Baked Stuffed Squash

The easiest way prepare squashes is to slice, seed, and bake cut-side down in a little water until tender, then drizzle with maple syrup, brown sugar, or butter. Ready for something new? Try adding a filling.—AA.

2 medium acorn or butternut squash
Filling:
2 cups canned crushed pineapple, drained
3/4 cup raisins
3/4 cup chopped pecans
1 teaspoon cinnamon
1/2 cup shredded Cheddar cheese (about 2 ounces)

Preheat the oven to 350°. Cut the squash in half and remove the seeds. Place the squash cut-side down in a large baking pan filled with a half-inch of water. Bake for 30 to 40 minutes until tender when pierced with fork. Combine the filling ingredients in a large bowl. Remove the cooked squash from the oven. Drain the water. Fill the squash cavities with stuffing mixture and bake cut-side up for another 10 to 15 minutes.

Serves 4

Variations:
- Try other squashes, like spaghetti squash.
- Try other fillings: sauté chopped apples, raisins, sugar, and nutmeg in butter until the fruit is golden brown. Add a little orange juice and simmer until the fruit is tender, about 8 to 10 minutes, and fill the squash.
- Scoop out cooked squash from the peel and puree with butter, cream, cheese, sweeteners, juices and/or spices.

Tip: Slicing through squashes can be very difficult. Use a sharp, heavy knife and make sure the squash is steady. Push down on the knife or use a serrated knife and a saw-like motion.

Tip: Some stores now sell precut squash in bags.

Tip: Also try squash in soups, stews, and casseroles.

Tahini Dressing

This dressing is a staple in our refrigerator. We use it on everything:
grains, vegetables, and greens.—ST

1/2 cup soy sauce, or to taste
1/2 cup lemon juice
5 tablespoons tahini
1 teaspoon dill weed, dried
2 to 3 garlic cloves, crushed
1 cup extra-virgin olive oil

Blend all ingredients except the oil in blender. Drizzle in the oil a little at a time until well blended.

Serves 6 to 8

Variations:

- Try other types of oil.
- Look for quality soy sauce: try tamari, shoyu, or low-sodium soy sauce products.
- Try different herbs: basil, parsley, or thyme.

Tip: Tahini is a ground sesame paste found in tubes or jars (similar to nut butters). It is available in some supermarkets and most health food stores.

Tip: Look for other sauce recipes. They can be enticements for picky eaters.

Tip: Use extra tahini to make hummus (bean dip with chickpeas, tahini, garlic, and olive oil).

Snacks and Desserts: Quick Ideas

Snacks typically refer to smaller portions of foods eaten between meals, while desserts, usually served after dinner, tend to be sweet treats. Try equating "snacks and desserts" with nutritious foods rather than something sweet. If you have dessert every night, try shifting to fruit with a little something sweet (cream, ice cream, or frozen yogurt) or simply plain fruit. Save sweet desserts for weekends or special occasions such as birthdays and holidays.

<u>Trail Mix:</u> Dried fruit, nuts, and whole-grain cereal, one of the easiest snacks. There are so many varieties to choose from: raisins, apricots, figs, almonds, cashews, walnuts, and a favorite, enticing cereal or granola. Put in a few dark chocolate chips if desired.

<u>Whole Grain Breads and Toppings:</u> Thick breads, quick breads, crackers, or pitas topped with a favorite cheese, nut butter, hummus, or other spread make a great treat. Hummus, a bean dip made with chickpeas, olive oil, garlic, and tahini, is a popular choice with vegetables or pita pieces. It is now available in many supermarkets, or make your own and omit the preservatives.

<u>Produce and Dips:</u> Try fruit and yogurt or nut butter; vegetables and a favorite salad dressing or bean dip. Use plain fruit for dessert or serve with a little cream or ice cream. And don't forget about baked fruits, such as apples and pears with cinnamon or nutmeg.

<u>Nachos with Salsa, Beans, and Cheese:</u> Find healthful chips and a natural salsa; top with beans and cheese for a nutritious treat.

<u>Frozen Treats:</u> MYO ice pops by freezing a favorite juice or smoothie. Look for quality all-natural ice creams, frozen yogurts, and sherbets. Frozen treats made with soy or rice milk are also available, as well as puddings and custards, but as with all products, watch for undesirable additives.

See also "Smoothies" in "Breakfasts."

Maple Zucchini Bread

Breads and muffins with vegetables rather than fruits tend to have lower glycemic loads. This recipe can interchange with carrots easily.—AA

1 1/2 cup unbleached all-purpose flour

1 cup whole-wheat flour

1 tablespoon baking powder

1 teaspoon cinnamon

1/4 teaspoon salt

8 tablespoons butter, melted or substitute 1/2 cup oil

3 eggs

1 cup maple syrup

1 teaspoon vanilla

1 1/2 cups shredded zucchini

1 cup walnuts, chopped

Preheat the oven to 350° and lightly coat 8 x 4-inch loaf pan with butter. In large bowl, mix together the flours, baking powder, cinnamon, and salt. Set aside. In a separate bowl, whisk together the butter, syrup, eggs, vanilla, and zucchini. Mix the wet ingredients into the dry ingredients. Stir until just blended. Fold in the walnuts. Pour the batter into the prepared loaf pan and bake for 1 hour, or until a knife inserted in the center comes out clean. Let cool for 5 to 10 minutes before removing from the pan.

Serves 4 to 6

Variations:

- Substitute yellow summer squash carrots for zucchini.
- Add zest of 1 lemon.
- Subsitue other types of nuts in place of walnuts.

Tip: Make a "master mix" of dry ingredients for quick, easy-to-make muffins or breads.

Tip: Make muffins and cut the cooking time in half.

Tip: Shred extra zucchini and freeze for later use.

Banana Molasses Bread

Here is a whole-grain variation on an old favorite. The molasses adds a source of iron.—ST

1 cup unbleached all-purpose flour, or spelt flour
1/2 cup whole-wheat flour
1/3 cup rolled oats
1 teaspoon baking soda
1 teaspoon cinnamon
1/2 teaspoon salt
2/3 cup sugar
4 tablespoons (1/2 stick) butter, at room temperature
1/3 cup blackstrap molasses
1 teaspoon vanilla extract
2 eggs
1 cup mashed ripe banana (2 to 3 medium bananas)
1/3 cup plain yogurt

Preheat the oven to 350° and lightly coat an 8 x 4-inch loaf pan with butter. In a medium bowl, whisk together the flours, oats, baking soda, cinnamon, and salt. In separate bowl combine the sugar, butter, molasses, and vanilla and beat until well blended. Add the eggs, banana, and yogurt and beat until well blended. Add in the flour mixture gradually and beat until just moistened. Pour the batter into the prepared loaf pan and bake for 1 hour, or until a knife inserted in the center comes out clean. Cool for 10 minutes on a rack and then remove from the pan.

Serves 4 to 6

Variations:
- Add 1/2 cup of chopped walnuts.
- Use a blend of unbleached all-purpose flour and other whole-grain flours for variety of nutrients and flavors.
- Buy "baking" bananas on sale. Peel and freeze for later use.

Tip: Make muffins and cut the cooking time in half.
Tip: For those with blood sugar problems, vegetable breads may be a better choice (pumpkin, carrot, or zucchini).

Apple Crisp

A classic dessert with many variations. Serve warm with a little vanilla ice cream.—AA

4 apples, peeled, cored and chopped
6 tablespoons of butter
2/3 cup rolled oats
1/3 cup whole-wheat pastry flour
1 teaspoon cinnamon
1/3 cup chopped walnuts

Preheat the oven to 375° and lightly coat an 8 x 8-inch baking dish with butter. Place the apples in the baking dish. Pulse the butter, oats, flour, and cinnamon in a food processor until lumpy (not smooth). Add the walnuts, pulse to mix, and pour the mixture on top of the apples. Bake for 20 to 30 minutes, or until lightly brown.

Serves 4 to 6

Variations:

- Use a blend of unbleached all-purpose flour and whole-wheat flour to ease the transition on taste buds. Slowly increase the amount of whole-wheat flour or other whole-grain flours for a variety of nutrients and flavors.
- Try other fruits such as berries, cherries, peaches, pears, and plums.
- Try other nuts such as almonds, which pair nicely with cherries.

Tip: When fresh fruit is unavailable, defrost frozen fruit in the refrigerator to use in a crisp that night for a little taste of summer in the winter.

Tip: Add small amounts of oil to moisten the topping mixture if it is too dry.

Tip: See also crumble, cobbler, and tart recipes made with fruits and whole grains. (For those with blood sugar problems, pumpkin pie may be a better choice. Pumpkin has a lower glycemic index than most fruits, and dairy ingredients help slow digestion.)

Carrot Cake

We had carrot cake for our wedding and use it as our standard
birthday cake. Pineapple and walnuts add moisture and crunch!
—AA

1 cup unbleached all-purpose flour

1/3 cup whole-wheat flour

1 cup sugar

1 teaspoon baking soda

1 teaspoon baking powder

2 teaspoons cinnamon

1/4 teaspoon nutmeg

1/2 teaspoon salt

2/3 cup oil

3 eggs

2 cups grated carrots

1 cup unsweetened crushed pineapple, drained

1/2 cup chopped walnuts

Preheat the oven to 350°. Grease and flour a 9 x 13-inch baking dish. Combine the flours, sugar, baking soda, baking powder, cinnamon, nutmeg, and salt in a large bowl. Add the oil and eggs. Stir well. Mix in the carrots, pineapple, and walnuts. Bake for 45 minutes or until a knife inserted in the center comes out clean. Let cool.

Serves 4 to 6

Variations:

- Substitute zucchini for carrots.
- Add 1 cup of raisins or other dried fruit.
- Substitute other nuts, such as pecans, for walnuts.
- Use 7/8 cup of honey instead of sugar (reduce the pineapple to 7/8 cup).

Tip: To make muffins, cut the cooking time in half.

Tip: Tastes great plain, or make a cream cheese frosting.

Tip: Mix extra pineapple with sweet potatoes and a dash of cinnamon for a side dish.

Apple Fig Bars

Fruit bar cookies are a nice break from traditional cookies and they make a wholesome, tasty snack.—AA

2 large apples, peeled, cored, and chopped
2 tablespoons lemon juice
2 tablespoons water
1 1/2 cup dried figs, chopped
1 cup (2 sticks) butter, softened
1 1/2 cup unbleached all-purpose flour
1 cup whole-wheat flour
1 cup sugar
1 cup chopped walnuts
1 teaspoon cinnamon
1 teaspoon salt

Preheat the oven to 375° and coat a 9 x 13 inch pan with butter. In a medium saucepan combine apples, lemon juice, and water. Simmer for 5 to 10 minutes, stirring occasionally until apples are tender. Add figs and stir for another 5 minutes mashing until puree turns smooth. Remove from heat and set aside. In large bowl mix remaining ingredients until well blended. Press half the mixture evenly into prepared pan and spread with the apple-fig puree. Crumble remaining flour mixture on top, pressing lightly. Bake for 35 to 40 minutes. Cool completely and cut into bars. Makes 2 dozen cookies

Variations:
- Substitute other dried fruit (apricots, dates, or prunes) for figs.
- Try sliced almonds in place of walnuts.
- Experiment with other whole-grain flours.

Tip: If bars tend to crumble, press layers together firmly before baking.
Tip: Look for other granola, cereal, and fruit bar recipes.
Tip: Bars can also be frozen.

Appendix A

Favorite Food List

This is a sampling of real foods to keep stocked in the pantry, refrigerator, or freezer. If possible, buy local, sustainable products. For those becoming familiar with products in stores, popular brands are listed. New products are constantly being brought to market. As always, read labels and look for real food ingredients.

Pantry

Whole grains: barley, millet, oats, quinoa, rice (Lundberg Farms, Bob's Red Mill)

Whole grain products: bread, cereal, crackers, pasta (Bionaturae, Deboles)

Vegetables and Fruits: avocados, garlic, potatoes, sweet potatoes, onions (separate from roots, their moisture causes sprouting), tomatoes, winter squash, bananas, citrus fruits, melons, and pineapple

Fruits (cans or jars): pineapple, olives, tangerines, applesauce, jams

Vegetables (cans or jars) : pumpkin, tomato products (Muir Glen)

Oils: coconut, olive, sesame, peanut (Spectrum Naturals)

Beans (canned): black, kidney, chick peas, white (Amy's, Eden, Westbrae)

Beans (dried): black, pinto, lentils, split peas

Seafood (canned): salmon, tuna, crab, anchovies

Sweets/Sweeteners: raw honey, maple syrup, maple sugar, molasses, dehydrated cane sugar juice (Sucanat, Rapa dura), cocoa powder, dark chocolate

Seasonings: sea salt, herbs, spices (Frontier, Herbamare, Penzeys)

Condiments: vinegars, stocks, soy sauce (tamari), Worcestershire sauce, mustard, ketchup, mayonnaise, dressings, salsa, pickles, olives

Refrigerator

Stone-ground whole-grain products: flour, pancake mix, hot cereal (Arrowhead Mills, Bob's Red Mill, Fiddler's Green)

Sprouted grain products: bread, bagels, tortillas (Pacific Bakery, Shiloh Farms)

Vegetables and Fruits: most vegetables, bag greens (Earthbound), dark leafy greens, lettuces, broccoli, carrots, celery, peppers, asparagus, ripe fruit (except bananas, citrus, melons, and pineapples), cut fruit, berries, and dried fruit (Pavich)

Nuts and seeds: almond, cashew, macadamia, walnut, pumpkin, sunflower

Nut butters: almond, cashew, peanut (Maranatha)

Flax Oil (Barlean's, Spectrum)

Hummus (Far East),

Tofu (Mori-Nu, White Wave)

Fresh fish

Yogurt (Stonyfield, Brown Cow)

Cheese (Organic Valley, Horizon)

Butter (Organic Valley)

Eggs

Poultry: chicken, turkey, and their products (sausages, hot dogs, ground)

Meat products: beef, pork, lamb, game meats

Processed meats: bacon, lunchmeat, hot dog (Applegate Farms, Shelton's)

Freezer

Surplus sprouted and whole grain bread products (Alvarado, Food for Life)

Vegetables and Fruit (Cascadian Farms, Sno-Pac); bananas (peeled, bagged)

Surplus nuts, seeds, butter, and some cheeses

Surplus fish, poultry, meats, and their products

Prepared foods: chicken nuggets, pizza, and other quality foods

Ice cream

Appendix B

Resources and Information for Food Groups

Grains

Glycemic Index

University of Sydney   www.glycemicindex.com

Information on the Glycemic Index (GI) of foods, latest GI data, GI books, GI testing services and information on the GI symbol program. (See also *The Glucose Revolution,* by Jennie Brand-Miller, Kaye Foster-Powell, and Johanna Burani.)

Gluten Intolerance Group (GIG)   (206) 246-6652

15110 10th Ave SW, Suite A   www.gluten.net
Seattle, WA 98166

Provides information, education, and support to persons with gluten intolerance diseases and their families, health care professionals, and the general public.

Bob's Red Mill Natural Foods, Inc.   (800) 349-2173

5209 SE International Way   www.bobsredmill.com
Milwaukee, OR 97222

Emphasizing stone ground whole grain products: grains, flours, cereals, mixes, seeds, beans, and more. Some products are available in stores. For more variety, shop online.

Fiddler's Green Farm   (800) 729-7935

P.O. Box 254   www.fiddlersgreenfarm.com
Belfast, ME 04915

Mail order organic, stone ground whole grains, whole grain flours, cereals, mixes (pancake, waffle, muffin, cookie, cakes), and more. Order by catalogue or shop online.

Hodgson Mill, Inc   (800) 525-0177
1203 Niccum Avenue   www.hodgsonmill.com
Effingham, IL 62401

Stone ground whole grain products. Some products are available in stores. Also, shop by catalogue or online.

Fruits and Vegetables

Environmental Working Group (EWG)
1436 U Street NW, Suite 100   (202) 667 – 6982
Washington, DC 20009   www.ewg.org

For information on pesticides and the "Shopper's Guide to Pesticides in Produce" visit their companion site at www.foodnews.org.

Alternative Farming Systems Information Center (AFSIC)
National Agricultural Library, Room 132
10301 Baltimore Ave.   (301) 504-6559
Beltsville MD 20705-2351   www.nal.usda.gov/afsic/

A resource at the National Agricultural Library provides information and links for defining and finding Community Supported Agricultural (CSA).

Robyn Van En Center for CSA Resources
Wilson College, Fulton Center for Sustainable Living
1015 Philadelphia Ave.   (717) 264-4141
Chambersburg, PA 17201   www.csacenter.org

A good resource for information, resources, and directories of CSA.

US Department of Agriculture
                              www.ams.usda.gov/farmersmarkets/index.htm

Agricultural Marketing Services provides a national directory of farmers markets, facts, resources, and other information including a coloring book for kids.

Local Harvest   www.localharvest.org

Another resource for CSA farms, farmers markets, food coops, and more.

Diamond Organics   (888) ORGANIC (674-2642)

P.O. Box 2159   www.diamondorganics.com

Freedom, CA 95019

A whole line of mail-order organic products including produce. Shop by catalogue or online.

Nuts, Seeds, and Oils

Spectrum Organic Products, Inc.   (800) 995-2705

Petamula, CA 94954   www.spectrumorganics.com

Coconut Oil, Cod Liver Oil, and Fish Oil*

Dr. Joseph Mercola   www.mercola.com

Optimal Wellness Center

1443 W. Schaumburg Road

Schaumburg, Illinois 60194

Also poultry, dairy, beef, wild game, and other quality products available online.

Coconut Oil and Cod Liver Oil*

Radiant Life   (888) 593-8333

PO Box 2326   www.4radiantlife.com

Novato, CA 94948

Call for a catalogue or visit online for quality sources of these oils.

*Other options available in "Fish" section.

Legumes

Soy Alert, Weston A. Price Foundation   (202) 333-HEAL

PMB Box 106-380   www.westonaprice.org/soy/soy_alert.html

4200 Wisconsin Avenue, NW

Washington, DC 20016

Eden Foods, Inc.   1-888-441-EDEN (3336)
701 Tecumseh Rd.   www.edenfoods.com
Clinton, MI 49236
    Organic pasta, beans, tomatoes, condiments, and more. Available in stores or online.

Sweeteners

Rapunzel Pure Organics   (800) 238-8090
P.O. Box 3483   www.efoodpantry.com
Springfield, IL 62708

Books on Sugar
    Lick the Sugar Habit by Nancy Appleton. New York: Avery
        Publishing Group, 1996.
    Get the Sugar Out by Ann Louise Gittleman, Ph.D. New York:
Three River Press, 1996.
    The Sugar Addict's Total Recovery Program by Kathleen DesMaisons,
Ph.D. New York: Ballantine Books, 2000.

Fish

Cod Liver Oil and Fish Oil*   (888)234-5656
J. R. Carlson Laboratories, Inc.   www.carlsonlabs.com
15 College Drive
Arlington Heights, IL 60004
    *Other options available in "Nuts, Seeds, and Oils" section.

Vital Choice Seafood   1-800-60-VITAL (608-4825)
605 30th Street   www.vitalchoice.com
Anacortes, WA 98221 .
    On-line shopping for canned and fresh-frozen wild salmon as well
as other products.

The Green Guide Institute   (212) 598-4910
Prince Street Station   www.thegreenguide.com
P.O. Box 567
New York, NY 10012

The Green Guide list to "Best Fish Picks" is available at their web site by subscription.

Environmental Working Group (EWG)   (202) 667–6982
1436 U Street NW, Suite 100   www.ewg.org
Washington, DC 20009
Information on PCBs and mercury in fish as well as a fish list for sensitive populations.

Monterey Bay Aquarium   (831) 648-4800
886 Cannery Row   www.montereybayaquarium.org
Monterey, CA 93940
Information to protect and restore ocean communities

The Audubon Society   (212) 979-3000
Audubon Action   www.seafood.audubon.org
1150 Connecticut Ave., NW, Suite 600
Washington, DC 20036

Blue Ocean Institute   (877) BOI-SEAS
250 Lawrence Hill Road   www.blueoceaninstitute.org
Cold Spring Harbor, NY 11724

Poultry and Eggs

Applegate Farms   (866) 587-5858
10 County Line Rd. #22   www.applegatefarms.com
Branchburg, NJ 08876
Natural and organic chicken, turkey, beef, and pork.

Shelton's Poultry, Inc   (800) 541- 1833
204 N. Loranne   www.sheltons.com
Pomona, CA 91767

Eat Well Guide   www.eatwellguide.org
An online directory for sustainable alternatives to factory farmed meat compiled by IATP and GRACE.

Eat Wild: The Clearinghouse for Information about Pasture-Based Farming
29428 129th Ave SW.   www.eatwild.com

Vashon WA 98070

Provides information about the benefits of pasture-based farming for animals, farmers, the environment, and our health. It has a link to a state-by-state directory for purchasing pasture-fed animal products.

West Wind Farms   (423) 965-3334
155 Shekinah Way   www.grassorganic.com
Deer Lodge, TN 37726

Organic, grass-fed chicken, turkey, lamb, beef, and dairy products.

Dairy

A Campaign for Real Milk   (202) 333-HEAL
Weston A. Price Foundation   www.realmilk.com
PMB Box 106-380
4200 Wisconsin Avenue, NW
Washington, DC 20016

Information and resource for raw milk and raw milk products.

Eat Wild: The Clearinghouse for Information about Pasture-Based Farming
29428 129th Ave SW.   www.eatwild.com
Vashon WA 98070

Provides information about the benefits of pasture-based farming for animals, farmers, the environment, and our health. It has a link to a state-by-state directory for purchasing pasture-fed animal products.

The Humane Society US
200 L Street, NW   www.hsus.org.
Washington, DC 20037

Write for a list of producers and distributors who pledge not to use RBGH.

Meyenberg Goat Milk Products   (800) 891-GOAT
PO Box 934   www.meyenberg.com
Turlock, CA 95381

Organic Consumers Association

www.organicconsumers.org/rBGH/rbghlist.cfm

Provides a list of RBGH-free suppliers, organic and nonorganic.

The Osteoporosis Education Project   (315) 432-1676

605 Fraklin Park Drive   www.betterbones.com

East Syracuse, NY 13057

Information on osteoporosis, acid / alkaline balance, as well as an acid / alkaline food chart.

Meats

Eat Wild: The Clearinghouse for Information about Pasture-Based Farming   www.eatwild.com

29428 129th Ave SW.

Vashon WA 98070

Provides information about the benefits of pasture-based farming for animals, farmers, the environment, and our health. It has a link to a state-by-state directory for purchasing pasture-fed animal products.

Grassland Beef   (877) 383-0051

R.R. 1, Box 20   www.grasslandbeef.com

Monticello, MO 63457

Eat Well Guide   www.eatwellguide.org

An online directory for sustainable alternatives to factory farmed meat compiled by IATP and GRACE.

Dr. Joseph Mercola   www.mercola.com

Optimal Wellness Center

1443 W. Schaumburg Road

Schaumburg, Illinois 60194

Poultry, dairy products, beef, wild game, and other quality products.

Herbs and Spices

Penzeys Spices   (800) 741-7787

19300 West Janacek Court   www.penzeys.com

PO Box 924

Brookfield, WI 53008

Appendix C
Resources for Sustainable Food Production and Food Cooperatives

US Department of Agriculture

www.ams.usda.gov/farmersmarkets

Agricultural Marketing Services Farmers Markets provides a directory and other information and the Alternative Farming Systems Information Center (AFSIC) at the National Agricultural Library provides links to organic food production, sustainable agriculture, and CSA farms at www.nal.usda.gov/afsic/.

Global Resource Action Center for the Environment
(GRACE) (212) 726-9161
215 Lexington Avenue, Suite 1001 www.factoryfarm.org
New York, NY 10016

Working to oppose factory farming and to promote sustainable food production that is healthful and humane, economically viable, and environmentally sound. Visit their site www.sustainabletable.org for healthy, sustainable food choices and www.eatwellguide.com compiled in collaboration with IATP for sustainable meat products (and do NOT miss their animated movie "The Meatrix," a "must-see!")

Institute for Agriculture and Trade Policy (IATP)
2105 First Avenue South (612) 870-3423
Minneapolis, MN, 55404 www.iatp.org

Promotes sustainable family farms, rural communities and ecosystems around the world through research and education, science and technology, and advocacy. See also the Eat Well Guide at www.eatwellguide.org.

Robyn Van En Center for CSA Resources
Wilson College, Fulton Center for Sustainable Living
1015 Philadelphia Ave.   (717) 264-4141 ext.3352
Chambersburg, PA, 17201   www.csacenter.org

Local Harvest   www.localharvest.org
    A resource for CSA farms, farmers markets, food coops, and more

Coop Directory Service: Find a Natural Food Coop Near You
1254 Etna Street   (651) 774-9189
St. Paul, MN 55106   www.coopdirectory.org
    Learn about food cooperatives, buying clubs, and distributors.
What they are, how to find one, or how to start one.

Resources for Organic Information and Products

USDA National Organic Program   (202) 720-3252
Room 4008 S. Bldg., Ag Stop 0268   www.usda.gov/nop
1400 Independence, SW
Washington, DC 20250
    Explain the national standards for the organic food labeling
program as well as other information.

Environmental Working Group (EWG)   (202) 667–6982
1436 U Street NW, Suite 100   www.ewg.org
Washington, DC 20009
    A not-for-profit environmental research organization dedicated
to improving public health and protecting the environment by reducing pollution in the air, water, and food. For information on pesticides in produce visit their site www.foodnews.org.

The Green Guide Institute   (212) 598-4910
Prince Street Station   www.thegreenguide.com
P.O. Box 567
New York, NY 10012

A non-profit research and education organization which provides environmental and health information for consumers. Available via newsletter or the web by subscription.

Organic Trade Association (OTA)   (413) 774-7511
PO Box 547   www.ota.com
Greenfield, MA 01302

A membership-based trade association for the organic industry. Search for products, services, and other information at www.theorganicreport.com.

Organic Consumers Association (OCA)   (218) 226-4164
6101 Cliff Estate Road   www.organicconsumer.org
Little Marais, MN 55614

A non-profit organization focused on issues of food safety, industrial agriculture, genetic engineering, corporate accountability, and environmental sustainability.

Health Care Professionals

The American Association of Naturopathic Physicians
3201 New Mexico Avenue, NW Suite 350   (866) 538-2267
Washington, DC 20016   www.naturopathic.org

American College for Advancement in Medicine (ACAM)
23121 Verdugo Drive, Suite 204   (800)532-3688
Laguna Hills, CA 92653   www.acam.org

National Association of Nutrition Professionals (NANP)
PO Box 971   (800) 342-8037
Veradale, WA 99037   www.nanp.org

Other Interesting and Helpful Web Sites

Slow Foods USA   (212) 965-5640
434 Broadway, 6th Floor   www.slowfoodusa.org
New York, NY 10013

A movement begun in Italy in 1986 to help counteract the fast food mentality, Slow Food USA is a non-profit educational organization dedicated to supporting and celebrating the food traditions of North America.

Equipment

Cold packs (wide variety of non-toxic ice packs)

Cold Ice, Inc.	(800) 525-4435
9999 San Leandro St	www.coldice.com
Oakland, CA 94603	

Grain Grinders

Radiant Life	(888) 593-8333
PO Box 2326	www.4radiantlife.com
Novato, CA 94948	

Kid-size Equipment

Betty Crocker	(800) 432-4959
P.O. Box 1118	www.bettycrocker.com
Minneapolis, MN 55440	

Small World Toys	
5711 Buckingham Parkway	(866) 310-1717
Culver City, CA 90230	www.smallworldtoys.com

Thermos (stainless-steel, small, wide mouth)

Gold Mine Natural Food Company	
7805 Arjons Drive	(800) 475-FOOD
San Diego, CA 92126-4368	www.goldminenaturalfood.com

Cooking and Recipe Web Sites

www.allrecipes.com
www.culinary.net
www.foodandhealing.com
www.kitchenlink.com
www.cooks.com
www.epicurious.com
www.whfoods.org

Appendix D

Recommended Reading

Health and Nutrition Books:

Better Bones, Better Body by Susan E. Brown. Ph.D. Los Angeles: Keats Publishing, 2000. (See also informaton from the Osteoporosis Education Project at www.betterbones.com)

Eat, Drink and Be Healthy by Walter C. Willet, M.D. New York: Fireside, 2001.

Eating Well for Optimal Health by Andrew Weil, M.D. New York: Alfred A Knopf, 2000. (Other books by Dr. Weil: *8 Weeks to Optimal Health* and *The Healthy Kitchen* with Rosie Daily. Also visit his web site Ask Dr. Weil www.drweil.com)

The Family Nutrition Book by William Sears, M.D., and Martha Sears, R.N. Boston: Little Brown and Company, 1999.

Healing with Whole Foods by Paul Pitchford. Berkeley, California: North Atlantic Books,1993. (Very intense, packed with information, initially overwhelming, but superior information when ready.)

Nourishing Traditions by Sally Fallon with Mary G. Enig, Ph. D. Washington, DC: New Trends Publishing, Inc., 2001. (May be initially overwhelming but thought provoking. See also *Nutrition and Physical Degeneration* by Weston A. Price, D.D.S. and the Weston A. Price Foundation at www.westonpricefoundation.org)

Pasture Perfect: The Far-Reaching Benefits of Choosing Meat, Eggs, and Dairy Products from Grass-fed Animals by Jo Robinson. Vashon Island Press, Vashon, WA, 2004. (Also see her web site at www.eatwild. com.)

User's Guide to Calcium and Magnesium by Nan Kathryn Fuchs, Ph.D. North Bergen, NJ: Basic Health Publications, 2002.

The Whole Food Bible by Christopher Kilham. Rochester, Vermont: Healing Arts Press, 1997. (Great information and a good resource.)

Reference:

The New Whole Foods Encyclopedia by Rebecca Wood. New York : Penguin, 1999. (An A-Z reference guide for plant foods.)

Good Food: The Comprehensive Food and Nutrition Resource by Margaret M. Wittenberg. Freedom, CA: The Crossing Press, 1998.

Glycemic Index:

The Glucose Revolution by Jennie Brand-Miller, Jennie, Kaye Foster-Powell, and Johanna Burani. New York: Marlowe & Company, 2000. (A good resource for anyone battling diabetes or blood sugar problems. See also University of Sydney Glycemic Index web site www.glycemicindex.com)

Limiting Sugar:

Lick the Sugar Habit by Nancy Appleton. New York: Avery Publishing Group, 1996.

Get the Sugar Out by Ann Louise Gittleman. New York: Three River Press, 1996. (See other books by this author.)

The Sugar Addict's Total Recovery Program by Kathleen DesMaisons, Ph.D. New York: Ballantine Books, 2000.

Cookbooks:

The All New Joy of Cooking by Irma S. Rombauer, Marion Rombauer Becker and Ethan Becker. New York: Scribner, 1997.

Betty Crocker's Cookbook, New York: MacMillian, 1996. (See also *Betty Crocker's Cooking Basics* for more novice cooks.)

Eating Clean by Lisa Allen. Nashua, NH: Morning Glory Press, 2002.

Feeding the Whole Family by Cynthia Lair. Seattle, WA: Moon Smile Press, 1997.

Healthy Cooking for Kids by Shelly Null. New York: St. Martin's Griffin, 1999.

Healthy Foods by Leanne Ely. Fox Point, WI: Champion Press, LTD, 2001.

The Healthy Kitchen by Andrew Weil and Rosie Daley.

How to Cook Everything by Mark Bittman. New York: Macmillan, 1998. (See also *How to Cook Everything: the Basics* for more novice cooks.)

How to Cook Without a Book by Pam Anderson. New York: Broadway Books, 2000.

Saving Dinner: The Menus, Recipes, and Shopping Lists to Bring Your Family Back to the Table by Leanne Ely. New York: Ballantine Books, 2003.

Whole Foods for the Whole Family edited by Roberta Bishop Johnson, La Leche League International, 1993.

Interesting Reading:

The Crazy Makers: How the Food Industry Is Destroying Our Brains and Harming Our Children by Carol Simonacchi. J. P. Tarcher, 2001.

Fast Food Nation: The Dark Side of the All-American Meal by Eric Schlosser. New York: Houghton Mifflin, 2002. (Excellent read and excellent information - painstakingly documented book. Highly recommended.)

Food Politics: How the Food Industry Influences Nutrition and Health by Marion Nestle. Berkeley, CA: University of California Press, 2003.

Food Fight: The Inside Story of the Food Industry, Americas Obesity Crisis, and What We Can Do About It by Kelly D. Brownell and Katherine Battle Horgen. McGraw-Hill/Contemporary Books, 2003.

Parenting / Children:

Cooking Time is Family Time by Lynn Fredericks. New York: William Morrow and Company, 1999. (out of print – check your library.)

How to Talk So Kids Will Listen and Listen So Kids Will Talk by Adele Faber and Elaine Mazlish. New York: Avon, 1982. (a "must-have" resource for any parent.)

How to Get Your Kid to Eat But Not Too Much by Ellyn Satter. Boulder, CO: Bull Publishing, 1987.

Pretend Soup and Other Real Recipes by Mollie Katzen and Ann

Henderson. Berkeley, CA: Tricycle Press, 1994. (Also see Katzen's other book, Honest Pretzels, for older children.)

Super Baby Food by Ruth Yaron. Archbald, PA: F. J. Roberts Publishing Company, 1998. (Not just for babies - great resource.)

Superimmunity for Kids by Leo Galland, M. D . New York: Copestone Press, Inc., 1988.

Magazines:

Eating Well: The Magazine of Food and Health

823A Ferry Road   (800)337-0402
Charlotte, VT 05445   www.eatingwell.com

Great information, wonderful recipes, and beautiful photos. Try a sample issue and you'll be hooked.

Living Without   (847)480-8810
PO Box 2126   www.livingwithout.com
North brook, IL 60065

A lifestyle guide for people with allergies and food sensitivities.

Taste for Life   (603)924-7271
86 Elm Street
Peterborough, NH 03458

Complimentary magazine available in many health practitioners' offices and natural food stores.

Green Guide

The Green Guide Institute   (212) 598-4910
Prince Street Station   www.thegreenguide.com
P.O. Box 567

Bibliography:

Appleton, Nancy. Lick the Sugar Habit. *New York: Avery Publishing* Group, 1996.

Balch, Phyllis A. and *Balch, James F.* Prescription for Nutritional Healing (3rd edition). *New York: Avery Penguin Putnam, 2000.*

Balch, Phyllis A. Prescription for Dietary Wellness. *New York: Avery Publishing Group, 1998.*

Brand-Miller, Jennie, Kaye Foster-Powell, and Johanna Burani, The Glucose Revolution, *New York: Marlowe & Company, 2000.*

Brown, Susan E. Better Bones, Better Body. *Los Angeles: Keats Publishing, 2000.*

Brownell, Kelly D. and Katherine Battle Horgen. Food Fight: The Inside Story of the Food Industry, Americas Obesity Crisis, and What We Can Do About It. *McGraw-Hill/Contemporary Books, 2003.*

Colbin, Annemarie. The Book of Whole Meals. *New York: Ballantine Books, 1983.*

Crayhon, Robert. Robert Crayhon's Nutrition Made Simple. *New York: M. Evans and Company, Inc., 1994.*

Fallon, Sally with Mary G. Enig. Nourishing Traditions. *Washington, DC: New Trends Publishing, Inc., 2001.*

Fredericks, Lynn. Cooking Time is Family Time. *New York: William Morrow and Company, 1999.*

Fuchs, Nan Kathryn. User's Guide to Calcium and Magnesium. *North Bergen, NJ: Basic Health Publications, 2002.*

Galland, Leo. Superimmunity for Kids. *New York: Copestone Press, Inc., 1988.*

Gittleman, Ann Louise. Get the Sugar Out. *New York: Three River Press, 1996.*

Gittleman, Lousie. Eat Fat, Lose Weight. *Los Angeles: Keats Publishing, 1999.*

Kilham, Christopher S. The Whole Food Bible. *Rochester, Vermont: Healing Arts Press, 1997.*

Kimbrell, Andrew (editor). The Fatal Harvest Reader. *Washington: Island Press, 2002.*

Mazlish, Elaine and Adele Faber. How to Talk So Kids Will Listen and Listen So Kids Will Talk. *New York: Avon, 1982.*

Nestle, Marion. Food Politics: How the Food Industry Influences Nutrition and Health. *Berkeley, CA: University of California Press, 2003.*

Null, Shelly. Healthy Cooking for Kids. New York: *St. Martin's Griffin, 1999.*

Pirello, Christine. Cooking the Whole Foods Way. *New York: HP-Books, 1997.*

Pitchford, Paul. Healing with Whole Foods. *Berkeley, California: North Atlantic Books, 1993.*

Price, Weston A. Nutrition and Physical Degeneration. *Weston A. Price, D.D.S., Keats Publishing 1997.*

Roberts, Susan B., and Heyman, Melvin B. Feeding Your Child for Lifelong Health. *New York: Bantam Books, 1999.*

Robinson, Jo. Pasture Perfect: The Far-Reaching Benefits of Choosing Meat, Eggs, and Dairy Products from Grass-fed Animals. *Vashon Island Press, Vashon, WA, 2004.*

Roehl, Evelyn. Whole Food Facts. *Rochester, Vermont: Healing Arts Press, 1996.*

Satter, Ellyn. How to Get Your Kid to Eat But Not Too Much. *Boulder, CO: Bull Publishing, 1987.*

Schlosser, Eric. Fast Food Nation: The Dark Side of the All-American Meal. *New York: Houghton Mifflin, 2002.*

Schmidt, Michael A. Brain-Building Nutrition: The Healing Power of Fats & Oils. *Berkeley, CA: Frog, Ltd., 2001.*

Schwarzbein, Diana, and Deville, Nancy. The Schwarzbein Principle. *Deerfield, FL: Health Communications, Inc., 1999.*

Sears, William and Sears, Martha. The Family Nutrition Book. *Boston: Little Brown and Company, 1999.*

Weil, Andrew, M.D. Eating Well for Optimum Health. *New York: Alfred A. Knopf, 2000.*

Weil, Andrew, M.D. Eight Weeks To Optimum Health. *New York: Alfred A. Knopf, 1997.*

Weil, Andrew, M.D. and Rosie Daley. The Healthy Kitchen. *New York: Alfred A. Knopf, 2003.*

Willet, Walter C. Eat, Drink and Be Healthy. *New York: Fireside, 2001.*

Wittenberg, Margaret M. Good Food: The Comprehensive Food and Nutrition Resource. *Freedom, CA: The Crossing Press, 1998.*

Wood, Rebecca. The New Whole Foods Encyclopedia. *New York: Penguin, 1999.*

Yaron, Ruth. Super Baby Food. *Archbald, PA: F. J. Roberts Publishing Company, 1998.*

About the Authors

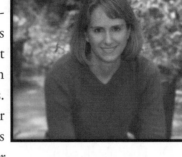

Allison Anneser is a New Hampshire-based writer whose work focuses on health and nutrition. After eight years of research and experience in managing personal health issues, Ms. Anneser ultimately incorporated her knowledge and successful strategies into *Refined to Real Food: Moving Your Family Toward Healthier, Wholesome Eating.*

A certified teacher with thirteen years of experience, Ms. Anneser works extensively with children, parents, and the community. She speaks frequently at libraries, schools, and other family-oriented organizations and has appeared on local and national radio and television programs.

Allison Anneser is a member of various parenting groups, the Society of Children's Book Writer's and Illustrators, and serves as a Regional Representative for the National Association of Women Writers. She resides in southern New Hampshire with her husband and two children. For more information, visit www.allisonanneser.com.

Dr. Sara Thyr is a naturopathic doctor who has helped
hundreds of people to experience
better health by altering their
eating habits. She has expertise in
nutrition and lifestyle counseling
and works to provide motivation
that people need to make important changes.

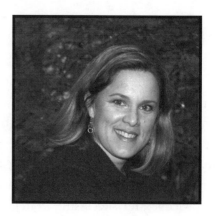

Dr. Thyr obtained her
naturopathic medicine and midwifery degrees at Bastyr University
in Kenmore, Washington. She was the first licensed naturopathic midwife in New Hampshire. She is currently serving on the
Naturopathic Board of Examiners and is the past-president of the
New Hampshire Association of Naturopathic Doctors. She is the
president of the American College of Naturopathic Obstetrics, and
is a member of the American Association of Naturopathic Midwives,
the American Association of Naturopathic Physicians, and the New
Hampshire Midwifery Association. She graduated cum laude from
Ottawa University in Ottawa, Kansas with a BA in Biology.

Dr. Thyr practices in Manchester and Concord, NH where she
specializes in women's health, infertility, pediatrics, and midwifery.
She sees patients with a wide range of illnesses, from common com-
plaints to serious digestive problems. When not attending to her busy
practice, Dr. Thyr enjoys cooking, gardening, tennis, bicycling and
swimming.

For more information or to contact Dr. Thyr, please visit her
website: www.DrThyr.com.